T0227244

Toxicologic Disorders

Editor

MEGAN C. ROMANO

VETERINARY CLINICS OF NORTH AMERICA: EQUINE PRACTICE

www.vetequine.theclinics.com

Consulting Editor
RAMIRO E. TORIBIO

April 2024 • Volume 40 • Number 1

ELSEVIER

1600 John F. Kennedy Boulevard • Suite 1800 • Philadelphia, Pennsylvania, 19103-2899

http://www.vetequine.theclinics.com

VETERINARY CLINICS OF NORTH AMERICA: EQUINE PRACTICE Volume 40, Number 1
April 2024 ISSN 0749-0739, ISBN-13: 978-0-443-12147-0

Editor: Taylor Hayes
Developmental Editor: Akshay Samson

Veterinary Clinics of North America: Equine Practice (ISSN 0749-0739) is published in April, August, and December by Elsevier Inc., 360 Park Avenue South, New York, NY 10010-1710. Business and Editorial Offices: 1600 John F. Kennedy Blvd., Suite 1800, Philadelphia, PA 19103-2899. Subscription prices are $314.00 per year (domestic individuals), $100.00 per year (domestic students/residents), $358.00 per year (Canadian individuals), $391.00 per year (international individuals), $100.00 per year (Canadian students/residents), and $180.00 per year (international students/residents). For institutional access pricing please contact Customer Service via the contact information below. To receive student/resident rate, orders must be accompanied by name of affiliated institution, date of term, and the signature of program/residency coordinator on institution letterhead. Orders will be billed at individual rate until proof of status is received. Foreign air speed delivery is included in all *Clinics* subscription prices. All prices are subject to change without notice. **POSTMASTER:** Send address changes to *Veterinary Clinics of North America: Equine Practice*, 3251 Riverport Lane, Maryland Heights, MO 63043. Customer Service (orders, claims, online, change of address): Elsevier Health Sciences Division, Subscription **Customer Service, 3251 Riverport Lane, Maryland Heights, MO 63043. Tel: 1-800-654-2452 (U.S. and Canada); 314-447-8871 (outside U.S. and Canada). Fax: 314-447-8029. E-mail: journalscustomerservice-usa@elsevier.com (for print support);** E-mail: **journalsonlinesupport-usa@elsevier.com (for online support)**.

Reprints. For copies of 100 or more of articles in this publication, please contact the Commercial Reprints Department, Elsevier Inc., 360 Park Avenue South, New York, NY 10010-1710. Tel.: 212-633-3874; Fax: 212-633-3820; E-mail: reprints@elsevier.com.

Veterinary Clinics of North America: Equine Practice is covered in *MEDLINE/PubMed (Index Medicus), Excerpta Medica, Current Contents/Agriculture, Biology and Environmental Sciences,* and *ISI.*

Contributors

CONSULTING EDITOR

RAMIRO E. TORIBIO, DVM, MS, PhD
Diplomate, American College of Veterinary Internal Medicine; Professor and Trueman
Endowed Chair of Equine Medicine and Surgery, College of Veterinary Medicine, The Ohio
State University, Columbus, Ohio

EDITOR

MEGAN C. ROMANO, DVM
Diplomate American Board of Veterinary Toxicology; Assistant Professor, Department of
Veterinary Science, Martin-Gatton College of Agriculture, Food, and Environment, Clinical
Toxicologist, University of Kentucky Veterinary Diagnostic Laboratory, University of
Kentucky, Lexington, Kentucky

AUTHORS

KARYN BISCHOFF, DVM, MS, MPH
Diplomate, American Board of Veterinary Toxicology; Associate Professor of Practice,
Department of Population Medicine and Diagnostic Sciences, Cornell University College
of Veterinary Medicine, New York State Animal Health Diagnostic Center, Ithaca, New
York

LYNNE CASSONE, DVM
Diplomate American College of Veterinary Pathologists; Diagnostic Pathologist, Veterinary
Diagnostic Laboratory, University of Kentucky, Lexington, Kentucky

SAVANNAH CHARNAS, DVM, MPH
Veterinary Toxicology Resident, Kansas State Veterinary Diagnostic Laboratory,
Manhattan, Kansas

T. ZANE DAVIS, PhD
Research Toxicology Scientist, USDA/ARS Poisonous Plant Research Laboratory, Logan,
Utah

STEVE ENSLEY, DVM, PhD
Clinical Veterinary Toxicologist, Kansas State Veterinary Diagnostic Laboratory,
Manhattan, Kansas

TIM J. EVANS, DVM, MS, PhD
Diplomate American College of Theriogenology; Diplomate American Board of Veterinary
Toxicology; Associate Professor, Department of Biomedical Sciences, College of
Veterinary Medicine and MU Extension, MU State Extension Specialist in Animal Health
and Veterinary Toxicology, University of Missouri, Columbia, Missouri

EMILY FINLEY, DVM
Postdoctoral Research Associate, Iowa State University College of Veterinary Medicine, Veterinary Diagnostic and Production Animal Medicine, Ames, Iowa

SCOTT A. FRITZ, DVM
Diplomate of the American Board of Veterinary Toxicology; Veterinary Toxicologist, Kansas State Veterinary Diagnostic Laboratory, Clinical Assistant Professor of Toxicology, Department of Anatomy and Physiology, Kansas State University College of Veterinary Medicine, Manhattan, Kansas

LYNDI L. GILLIAM, DVM, PhD
Diplomate of the American College of Veterinary Internal Medicine- Large Animal; Professor, Equine Internal Medicine, College of Veterinary Medicine, Oklahoma State University, Stillwater, Oklahoma

JEFFERY O. HALL, DVM, PhD
Diplomate of the American Board of Veterinary Toxicology; Technical Service Veterinarian for the Cattle Team at Huvepharma, Cattle Technical Services, Huvepharma Inc., Peachtree City, Georgia

STEPHEN B. HOOSER, DVM, PhD
Diplomate and Past-President of the American Board of Veterinary Toxicology; Professor of Toxicology and Head, Toxicology Section, Department of Comparative Pathobiology, Animal Disease Diagnostic Laboratory, College of Veterinary Medicine, Purdue University, West Lafayette, Indiana

LYNN ROLLAND HOVDA, RPH, DVM, MS
Diplomate, American College of Veterinary Internal Medicine; Director, Veterinary Medicine, Safetycall International and Pet Poison Helpline, Bloomington, Indiana; Adjunct Professor, Department of Veterinary and Biomedical Sciences, College of Veterinary Medicine, University of Minnesota, St Paul, Minnesota

MICHELLE MOSTROM, DVM, MS, PhD
Diplomate American Board Veterinary Toxicology; Diplomate American Board Toxicology (1995–2020); Veterinary Toxicologist, North Dakota State University, Veterinary Diagnostic Laboratory, Fargo, North Dakota

SCOTT RADKE, DVM, MS
Diplomate, American Board Veterinary Toxicology; Clinical Assistant Professor, Iowa State University College of Veterinary Medicine, Veterinary Diagnostic and Production Animal Medicine, Ames, Iowa

MEGAN C. ROMANO, DVM
Diplomate American Board of Veterinary Toxicology; Assistant Professor, Department of Veterinary Science, Martin-Gatton College of Agriculture, Food, and Environment, Clinical Toxicologist, University of Kentucky Veterinary Diagnostic Laboratory, University of Kentucky, Lexington, Kentucky

BEATRICE SPONSELLER, DVM
Diplomate, American Board of Veterinary Practitioners (Equine); Clinical Professor, Department of Veterinary Clinical Sciences, College of Veterinary Medicine, Iowa State University, Ames, Iowa

BRYAN L. STEGELMEIER, DVM, PhD
Veterinary Pathologist, USDA/ARS Poisonous Plant Research Laboratory, Logan, Utah

Contents

> Incidences of feed contamination are rare even though enormous amounts of animal feed are manufactured. However, there are still some cases of feed–related illness in horses. Veterinarians play a crucial role in recognizing and mitigating these events and in assessing the severity of risks. Due to these risks, proper reporting and consultation with government and state agencies are crucial. Accurate diagnosis and identification of the source of poisoning are promising when a thorough case workup is performed and agencies such as veterinary diagnostic laboratories and the US Food and Drug Administration Center for Veterinary Medicine are used effectively.

> This article is intended to highlight toxicosis-associated pathology in horses that might be observed by a clinician in the living animal and at gross necropsy. When the clinician is aware of these pathologic changes (particularly when coupled with a suggestive environmental or herd history), then collaboration with a diagnostic laboratory can begin to help identify specific toxicants. Proper sampling and communication with the diagnostic laboratory will vastly improve the likelihood of a specific diagnosis; postmortem sampling and specimen submission are reviewed in the last section of this article.

> Range and pasture toxic plants can poison horses. Many of these plants are noxious weeds that can dominate plant populations and replace healthy forages. Poisoning is often difficult to diagnose as the resulting plant-induced disease is similar to other infectious, toxic, and nutritional diseases. Identifying potentially problem plants, and observing what plants horses are eating, is essential in determining the risk of poisoning. If the risk is significant, it can drive management to invest in strategies to avoid exposure, animal disease, and suffering.

diarrhea, and liver damage but can be dramatic with neurologic signs associated with equine leukoencephalomalacia and tremorgens. Specific antidotes for mycotoxicosis are rare, and treatment involves stopping the use of contaminated feed, switching to a "clean" feed source, and providing supportive care.

Toxigenic Endophyte–Infected Tall Fescue and Ergot Alkaloids

Tim J. Evans and Megan C. Romano

"Fescue toxicosis" and reproductive ergotism present identical toxidromes in late-gestational mares and, likely, other equids. Both toxic syndromes are caused by ergopeptine alkaloids (EPAs) of fungal origin, and they are collectively referred to as equine ergopeptine alkaloid toxicosis (EEPAT). EPAs are produced by either a toxigenic endophyte (*Epichloë coenophiala*) in tall fescue and/or a nonendophytic fungus (*Claviceps purpurea*), infecting small grains and grasses. EEPAT can cause hypoprolactinemia-induced agalactia/dysgalactia, prolonged gestation, dystocia, and other reproductive abnormalities in mares, as well as failure of passive transfer in their frequently dysmature/overmature/postmature foals. Prevention relies on eliminating exposures and/or reversing hypoprolactinemia.

Cantharidin

Karyn Bischoff

Cantharidin is the toxic component of blister beetles of the genus *Epicauta*. Cantharidin is a potent vesicant which causes blisters, erosions, and ulcerations in the gastrointestinal and urinary tracts, and can cause myocardial necrosis. Blister beetles are found over most of North America and specifically contaminate alfalfa at harvest. History of alfalfa feeding, with colic, dysuria, hypocalcemia, and hypomagnesemia are suggestive of blister beetle toxicosis. Myocardial damage causes increased serum cardiac troponin 1. Tentative diagnosis can be made by finding the beetles in feed or ingesta. Definitive diagnosis requires detection of cantharidin in urine or gastric contents. Treatment involves ending exposure, decreasing absorption, controlling pain, using gastroprotectants, and fluids and electrolyte replacement. Prognosis is guarded to poor.

Blue Green Algae

Scott A. Fritz, Savannah Charnas, and Steve Ensley

Blue green algae cyanotoxins have become increasingly more prevalent due to environmental, industrial, and agricultural changes that promote their growth into harmful algal blooms. Animals are usually exposed via water used for drinking or bathing, though specific cases related to equines are very limited. The toxic dose for horses has not been determined, and currently only experimental data in other animals can be relied upon to aid in case interpretation and treatment. Treatment is mostly limited to supportive care, and preventative control methods to limit exposures are more likely to aid in animal health until more research has been performed.

> Snakebite envenomation (SBE) in horses can have devastating outcomes. Tissue damage, cardiotoxicity, coagulopathy, and neurotoxicity can be concerns with SBE. Understanding the actions of venom components is important in developing a successful treatment plan. Antivenom is the mainstay of treatment. Long-term deleterious effects can occur including cardiac dysfunction and lameness.

> This article provides information on the toxicity of some therapeutic drugs, illicit drugs, and supplements. Medications in the therapeutic section are grouped into antibiotics, antipsychotic agents, bronchodilators, nonsteroidal anti-inflammatory drugs, opioids, and sedatives/tranquilizers. The section on illicit drugs and supplements provides information on more specific medications including commonly used or abused human medications and a few that are available only from Internet compounding pharmacies. Many drugs and supplements can be either therapeutic or illicit depending on the dosage and ultimate use of the horse. Some medications, however, are illicit no matter when and how they are administered.

> Ionophores are a class of polyether antibiotics that are commonly used as anticoccidial agents and growth promotants in ruminant diets. Ionophores transport ions across lipid membranes and down concentration gradients, which results in mitochondrial destruction, reduced cellular energy production, and ultimately cell death. Cardiomyocytes are the primary target in equine patients when exposed to toxic concentrations and the clinical disease syndrome is related to myocardial damage. Animals can survive acute exposures but can have permanent heart damage that may result in acute death at future time points. Animals that survive a poisoning incident may live productive breeding lives, but physical performance can be greatly impacted. Animals with myocardial damage are at risk of sudden death and pose a risk to riders.

> This article provides an overview of several agricultural and industrial toxicants that are most likely to be encountered by horses. Overviews include brief backgrounds of the agents in question, potential sources of intoxication, mechanisms of action, clinical signs, lesions, diagnostic considerations, and treatment options.

VETERINARY CLINICS OF NORTH AMERICA: EQUINE PRACTICE

SERIES OF RELATED INTEREST

Veterinary Clinics of North America: Food Animal Practice
https://www.vetfood.theclinics.com/

THE CLINICS ARE NOW AVAILABLE ONLINE!
Access your subscription at:
www.theclinics.com

Preface

"... and Toxic"

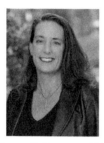

Megan C. Romano, DVM
Editor

Horses and other equids, like any other species, can be exposed to a variety of toxic substances. The true incidence of poisoning is difficult to estimate, and cases are likely underreported because there is no centralized mandatory reporting mechanism for poisoning in veterinary species. Such estimates rely on cases reported to poison control centers (eg, Pet Poison Helpline and ASPCA Animal Poison Control Center) or presented to referral hospitals. Underreporting is likely more severe in equines than in small animals, because equine practitioners and owners are less likely to call a poison control center than small animal practitioners and owners.

Unless the clinician has had prior experience, toxicant exposures are likely to be an afterthought in developing a differential diagnosis. Use of the "DAMN IT" mnemonic is apt to lead to a differential list that includes specific degenerative, anomalous, metabolic, neoplastic, and infectious diseases but which conclude with "and Toxic"—full stop. This issue aims to improve the practitioner's ability to diagnose and treat poisonings and envenomations. No toxicology text is comprehensive; because "the dose makes the poison," everything could theoretically be toxic. In addition, possible toxicoses and envenomations vary dramatically between different parts of the world, and this issue includes the most common/relevant toxic exposures encountered by equine practitioners in North America.

Diagnosing and managing toxic exposures can be challenging even for experienced practitioners. "Investigative and diagnostic toxicology and feed-related outbreaks" by Hooser and Wilson-Frank introduces general principles of investigative and diagnostic toxicology to assist the practitioner in identifying and narrowing down potential toxicologic differentials. This article also outlines the best approach to managing feed-related outbreaks. "Diagnostic pathology of equine toxicoses" by Cassone discusses antemortem and postmortem findings associated with certain toxic exposures in equines.

Vet Clin Equine 40 (2024) xi–xii
https://doi.org/10.1016/j.cveq.2023.12.003
0749-0739/24/© 2023 Published by Elsevier Inc.

The remaining articles are devoted to specific toxicants or classes of toxicants. Poisonous plant articles are organized based on their sources. "Plants that contaminate feed and forages and poison horses" by Stegelmeier covers plants that primarily cause problems when they contaminate feeds and forages. "Range and pasture plants likely to poison horses" by Stegelmeier introduces range and pasture plants that are typically ingested when better-quality forages are lacking. Plants that can cause myopathy if ingested in sufficient quantities are discussed in "Toxic myopathy plants (box elder, white snakeroot, and rayless goldenrod)" by Sponseller. Similarly, toxic garden and landscaping plants are introduced in "Toxic garden and landscaping plants" by Romano. "Pyrogallol toxicosis in horses" by Bischoff is specifically devoted to maples and *Pistacia* species.

"Equine Mycotoxins" by Ensley and Mostrom introduces various mycotoxins that can contaminate feeds and forages. "Toxigenic endophyte-infected tall fescue and ergot alkaloids" by Evans and Romano focuses on ergopeptine alkaloids in toxigenic endophyte-infected tall fescue grass and ergot fungus, both of which can affect grain-based feeds, pasture grasses, and hay. Blister beetles and cantharidin are discussed in "Cantharidin" by Bischoff. "Cyanobacteria (blue-green algae)" by Ensley, Fritz, and Charnas summarizes cyanotoxins and blue-green algae, and "Snake envenomation" by Gilliam focuses on snake envenomations. Therapeutic medications and even the most benign-appearing supplements can cause adverse effects under certain circumstances and are described in "Therapeutic medications and illicit medications and supplements" by Rolland Hovda. Ionophores, such as monensin, are discussed in "Ionophores" by Fritz and Hall. Finally, horses and other equids could potentially be exposed to various industrial and agricultural toxicants, which are covered in "Industrial and agricultural toxicants" by Radke and Finley.

I sincerely thank the authors, each an expert on their topic, for taking the time to contribute to this special issue of *Veterinary Clinics of North America: Equine Practice*. I am excited about it and proud of it, and I hope readers learn as much from reading it as I have learned editing it.

Megan C. Romano, DVM
Department of Veterinary Sciences
University of Kentucky
PO Box 14125
Lexington, KY 40512-4125, USA

E-mail address:
megan.romano@uky.edu

Investigation and diagnostic approaches

Investigative and Diagnostic Toxicology and Feed-Related Outbreaks

Stephen B. Hooser, DVM, PhD

KEYWORDS

- Feed-related • Poisoning • Investigation • Diagnostic testing • Reporting

KEY POINTS

- Outbreaks of feed contamination are rare but when they occur can affect multiple animals.
- The chances of an accurate diagnosis are increased if appropriate steps are taken from the outset of the investigation and if a veterinary toxicologist is on the team.
- Communications between the veterinarian and veterinary diagnostic laboratory are critical.
- It is important to report suspected cases of poisoning to ensure that the source is found, that other animals are not affected and that the feed is recalled if appropriate.

INTRODUCTION/BACKGROUND

There is the potential for horses to be exposed to a wide variety of poisons within their environment (**Fig. 1**). Fortunately, cases of feed-related poisoning are relatively rare. However, because incidents of contamination often occur in feed or commercially pre-pared forage, they can affect multiple animals simultaneously in one or more locations. Because some owners may only have one horse at their farm, it is important to report suspicions of feed-related poisoning so that isolated cases can be identified, grouped with other related cases, an investigation can be started, and the common cause of poisoning found and corrected (see "Reporting a suspected feed-related poisoning" sections in this chapter of this issue of Veterinary Clinics of North America [VCNA]) (**Figs. 2** and **3**).

Clinical signs of toxicosis in horses can vary greatly depending on the toxin/toxicant. The time from exposure to onset of clinical signs can also vary greatly depending on the toxin/toxicant, route of exposure, and dose. For example, accidental contamination and ingestion of feed with an ionophore such as monensin often results in the onset of adverse clinical signs within a short time following ingestion (see "Ionophores" by

Toxicology Section, Department of Comparative Pathobiology, Animal Disease Diagnostic Laboratory, College of Veterinary Medicine, Purdue University, 406 South University, West Lafayette, IN 47907, USA
E-mail address: shooser1@purdue.edu

Vet Clin Equine 40 (2024) 1–10
https://doi.org/10.1016/j.cveq.2023.12.001
0749-0739/24/© 2023 Elsevier Inc. All rights reserved.

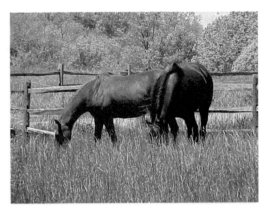

Fig. 1. Horses grazing in Boone Co, IN. (Horses in Boone County, Indiana. Norm Stephens. https://flic.kr/p/s1FxNj.)

Fritz and Hall in this issue of VCNA). In contrast, ingestion of the mycotoxin, aflatoxin, in feed more frequently results in the gradual onset of adverse clinical signs weeks to months after ingestion of sufficient amounts of contaminated feed (see "Mycotoxins" by Mostrom and Ensley in this issue of VCNA).

Adverse clinical signs related to cases of poisoning can affect one or multiple organ systems. Because of variability in clinical signs related to poisoning, time to onset of those signs, and individual variation, it is difficult to provide a comprehensive list of adverse clinical signs for each type of toxicosis. This is one of the many reasons it is of vital importance to have trained veterinary toxicologists in the diagnostic community. None-the-less, in many instances, suspicion of poisoning can be related to a recent change in feed, or feeding from a new lot of feed, followed by the appearance

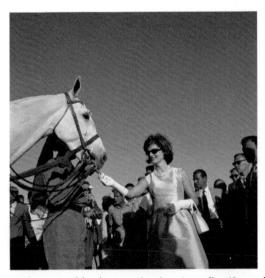

Fig. 2. Extremely unlikely cause of feed contamination. Jaqueline Kennedy Feeding a Horse. (Cecil Stoughton. White House Photographs. John F. Kennedy Presidential Library and Museum, Boston.)

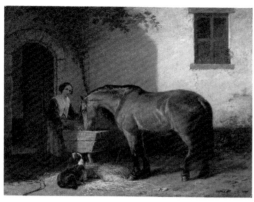

Fig. 3. Feeding the horse by Charles-Philogène Tschaggeny (Het voeren van het paard. Charles Philogène Tschaggeny. Brussel 1815-1894 Sint-Joost-ten-Node (België).)

of adverse clinical signs shortly thereafter, for example, in hours to days. An example of this would be the appearance of sweating, ataxia, and weakness within hours of ingestion of feed contaminated with monensin. Conversely, suspicion of feed-related poisoning can occur when animals present with gradual loss of weight and condition during an extended period, for example, from weeks to months, such as from chronic aflatoxin poisoning. Of course, it is important to remember that for some toxins, for example, aflatoxin, very high doses ingested during a short period can result in severe, acute liver damage within days, although in the case of aflatoxin, it is uncommon for horses to be exposed to high enough concentrations to cause acute toxicity.

Investigation of a Possible Case of Poisoning

To arrive at a diagnosis in a case of poisoning, the ideal situation is one where

1. The clinical syndrome, including historical information, clinical signs, and response to antidotal or appropriate therapy, is consistent with the suspected toxicant,
2. Pathologic and/or clinical pathologic findings are consistent with the suspected toxicant (see "Sample Collection" in "Diagnostic Pathology of Equine Toxicoses" by Cassone in this issue of VCNA),
3. There is a test, which indicates the biological effect of the suspected toxicant, and
4. Results of analytical testing confirm the presence of the suspected toxicant in the tissues of the patient at a level consistent with poisoning.

Obtaining as many of these facts as possible facilitates a diagnosis and requires communication and coordination among clients/owners, clinical veterinarians, and veterinary diagnosticians (eg, toxicologists and pathologists, toxicologists being absolutely essential).

NECROPSY AND GUIDELINES FOR SAMPLING
Collecting Appropriate Samples for Diagnostic Testing

After the case history is thoroughly documented, if there are deceased animals, establishing differential diagnoses should begin with a complete necropsy, if possible and diagnostic testing. Necropsy results can help refine the differential list and guide analytical testing, or in some cases can identify the causative agent, especially if the agent was a poisonous plant and can be identified in stomach contents. Therefore, collecting the appropriate samples from the affected animal(s) and saving as much of the suspect feed product as possible will be important in arriving at an accurate diagnosis. There are toxins which can only be identified in the feed that the animal was eating, such as most mycotoxins. Therefore, it is better to save too much than too little. As discussed in the following chapter, "Matthews refers to an unproven law that in this context predicts that the more certain the diagnostician is that no toxicant is involved, the more likely it will seem that intoxication has occurred. This probability increases in the direct proportion with the value of the horse and litigiousness of the owner and increases exponentially if inadequate samples for toxicologic testing are collected." (see "Sample Collection" in "Diagnostic Pathology of Equine Toxicoses" by Cassone in this issue of VCNA). If there are any questions regarding necropsy evaluation and sample collection, the veterinarian should contact their veterinary diagnostic laboratory for consultation and submission guidelines.

Moreover, it is very important to remember, if there is any suspicion that the horse died following ingestion of a toxic chemical, the carcass should never, ever be sent for rendering as some chemicals are not destroyed in the rendering process and can end up in various rendered products.

Establishing a Causal Relationship Between Clinical Signs and Suspect Foodstuff

Recent changes in feed that coincide chronologically with changes in the animal's eating behavior or with onset of adverse clinical signs can be suggestive of a food contamination issue. Obtaining a thorough case history is a critical first step in successfully establishing a causal relationship between the horse's clinical signs and the suspect feed source (**Box 1**). This will also help ascertain whether other differentials should be considered during the diagnostic workup of the case. Working in collaboration with the owner, the veterinarian should begin the case history at a point in time preceding the owner's first discovery that there was a problem and then progress chronologically from that point. A thorough case history should include detailed information about the animal(s) exposed as well as the feed product in question (**Box 2**). The following lists include important information that should be considered when taking the case history.

Box 1
Information regarding the animal exposed

1. Signalment (sex, breed, age, and weight of horse)
2. Horse's complete medical history (including vaccinations, medications, and treatments given)
3. Results of any diagnostic testing or clinical pathology testing performed (eg, complete blood count, chemistries, urinalysis, and serology)
4. Description of the progression of clinical signs (onset time, duration, and types of clinical signs exhibited)
5. Timeframe between feeding product and onset of clinical signs/change in behavior
6. Duration of exposure and approximate amount of feed product consumed
7. Number of horses affected at each location
8. Number of horses potentially exposed
9. Description of how the feed was stored/handled/delivered to farm
10. Consideration of other possibilities for source of exposure to other toxins/toxicants/drugs

---

Box 2
Regarding the feed product in question

1. Brand name of product and product description from the label

2. Type of feed product

3. Purchase date, purchase location, and total amount purchased

4. Type of product container (bag, feed bin, corn crib, and so forth)

5. Name of the manufacturer of the product

6. Lot number and expiration date (best by or best before date) if it is a commercial feed

7. UPC code (Universal Product Code = barcode)

8. Product date and product code

9. Amount of food product used and the amount the owner still has

10. Where and how the product was stored

The case information obtained by the veterinarian must be documented in case records with time and date. Once the case history and the information regarding the feed have been completed, the veterinarian can use the product information to query the FDA Center for Veterinary Medicine (CVM) food/feed recall products list. This can help to establish whether the food product in question has already been recalled due to contamination. The list of feed products recalled can be accessed at their website at: https://www.fda.gov/AnimalVeterinary/SafetyHealth/RecallsWithdrawals.

REPORTING A FEED COMPLAINT
Agencies Regulating Commercial Animal Feeds

The primary agencies regulating animal feeds are the US Food and Drug Administration (FDA) and the various state Association of American Feed Control Officials (AAFCO) laboratories. The AAFCO works in collaboration with the FDA to ensure the safety of commercial feeds. The AAFCO regulations on animal food products are intended to address the nutrient content of animal feeds and label claims on the product in an effort to guarantee uniform consistency and enforcement of these claims. The FDA's role involves regulating health claims on animal food products, particularly regarding the safety of new ingredients or feed additives. In 2007, the Food and Drug Administration Amendments Act was passed, giving the FDA more jurisdiction over taking action against animal feed contamination or safety issues. The FDA CVM is the primary authority for regulating health claims on feed labels. The Veterinary Laboratory Investigation and Response Network (Vet-LIRN) is a part of the FDA CVM, which responds to potential animal food issues and coordinates nonregulatory sampling and testing in a network of state veterinary diagnostic laboratories.[1]

How to Report a Feed Complaint

Veterinarians should not wait for diagnostic testing to be completed before reporting a suspected food-borne illness. If the practitioner has reasonable suspicion that the adverse health event was due to feed contamination, the veterinarian or owner can contact the manufacturer of the feed product. The manufacturer may be able to provide insight into the potential issue and will also need that information to trace increased occurrences associated with a particular product or ascertain if there is an outbreak associated with a specific geographic location. Subsequently, if the suspect feed is a commercial product, it may be appropriate to contact the state AAFCO laboratory to report a possible feed-related issue in order to initiate an investigation at the state level. If there is heightened suspicion that a contaminant in the feed is the source of illness (eg, diagnostic tests are completed at a veterinary diagnostic laboratory or a state AAFCO laboratory, or if most other differentials are eliminated), then the veterinarian should report an animal feed complaint to the FDA CVM. A complaint can be reported electronically through the FDA's "Safety Reporting Portal" or it can be reported by calling the FDA Consumer Complaint Coordinator in that state. By opening the FDA CVM website (https://www.safetyreporting.hhs.gov/), the "Safety Reporting Portal" can be accessed electronically and information regarding the clinical case history and food product can be entered. If reporting by telephone, the FDA CVM website (http://www.fda.gov/Safety/ReportaProblem/ConsumerComplaintCoordinators/) has an "FDA Consumer Complaint Coordinators" directory that lists the telephone number for the coordinators in each state. It is at this point that state veterinary diagnostic laboratories often begin working with the FDA CVM Vet-LIRN to coordinate collection of samples and testing if needed. In addition, once there is heightened suspicion of an animal toxicosis, it is often advisable to contact the State Veterinarian. In some states, there is a legal requirement to report some cases of animal poisoning, however this requirement, and the specific toxins/toxicants that must be reported, vary greatly from state to state.[1]

Reporting a Suspected Feed-Related Poisoning Through Your State Association of American Feed Control Officials Laboratory

The AAFCO is a nonprofit organization that sets standards for both animal feeds and pet foods in the United States. It helps to guide state and federal feed regulators. The members are charged by their state or federal laws to regulate the manufacture, sale, and distribution of animal feeds and animal drug remedies.[2]

Each state has an AAFCO member. However, individual states each have separate budgets, unique priorities and capabilities, and varying ability to investigate animal feed complaints. Some states have robust animal feed programs and, in many cases, can respond relatively quickly in the event of a suspected poisoning. For example, the Office of the Indiana State Chemist (OISC), the AAFCO laboratory for Indiana, makes sure that feeds are free from adulterants or contaminants and are properly labeled. OISC also administers laws regarding animal feeds to ensure feed safety. As such, it responds to owner complaints and concerns regarding the safety of feeds. In cases of animal illness, it works closely with the Animal Disease Diagnostic Laboratory at Purdue University to determine if feeds were contaminated or adulterated.

Reporting a Suspected Feed-Related Poisoning to the Food and Drug Administration

The FDA encourages horse owners, farmers, veterinarians, and other animal health professionals to report problems with feeds for livestock (including horses). Veterinarians or owners may report problems by either (1) submitting an electronic report using the Safety Reporting Portal or (2) calling your state's FDA Consumer Complaint Coordinator (**Fig. 4**).

It will facilitate entering the report if you have the following information available when submitting the complaint (**Box 3**).

If possible, please save the original packaging. The packaging contains IMPORTANT information often needed to identify the variety of food, the manufacturing plant,

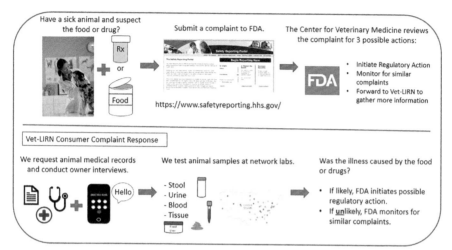

Fig. 4. What happens during a consumer complaint response? (Used with permission of the FDA CVM Vet-LIRN https://www.fda.gov/animal-veterinary/science-research/veterinary-laboratory-investigation-and-response-network.)

Box 3
Information needed for filing a report (a report may still be filed if some of the items cannot be obtained)[3]

Product information
1. Exact name of the product and product description (as stated on the product label)
2. Type of container (eg, bag, bale, block, bulk, drum, and so forth)
3. Lot number: This number is often hard to find and difficult to read. It is stamped onto the product packaging and typically includes a combination of letters and numbers, and is always in close proximity to the best by/before or expiration date (if the product has a best by/before or expiration date). The lot number is very important because it helps us determine the manufacturing plant as well as the production date.
4. Best by, best before, or expiration date
5. UPC code (Universal Product Code = bar code)
6. Net weight
7. Purchase date and location
8. Results of laboratory tests performed on the product or on the animals, if any
9. How the food was stored, prepared, and handled

Description of the problem with the product. Examples include the following:
1. Foul odor, off color, and inconsistent texture
2. Foreign material found in the product.

If you think animals have become sick or injured because of consuming a specific food, you may also provide information about the animals, including the following:
1. Species (Horse)
2. Age, weight, breed, production, pregnancy, lactation status, and housing
3. Previous health status of the animals including any known preexisting conditions
4. Other foods or drugs the animals received
5. Clinical signs observed (eg, diarrhea, lethargy, staggering, and so forth)
6. How soon after consuming the product the clinical signs appeared
7. If owner: Your veterinarian's or other consulted professional's contact information, diagnosis, and medical records
8. How many animals consuming the product were affected and how many were not
9. Why you suspect the product caused the illness

and the production date. For products delivered in bulk, information may be included on the bill of lading, receipt, or invoice.

DISCUSSION: HISTORICAL INCIDENTS OF FEED-RELATED POISONING IN HORSES

During the past 15 years, there have been several reported incidents of feed contamination, which have led to exposure, illness, or death of horses. In many of these instances, the contaminated feed was recalled from the marketplace. Recalls are actions taken by a firm to remove a product from the market. Recalls may be conducted on a firm's own initiative, by FDA request, or by FDA order under statutory authority.

Of these incidents, one contaminant that is associated with serious illnesses is the accidental contamination of batches of feed with the ionophore, monensin. Horses are particularly sensitive to the toxic effects, and monensin should never be incorporated into horse feed. One incident involving accidental contamination of feed with monensin resulted in 6 deaths with an additional 16 affected on one farm. In a separate incident, insufficient cleaning of a feed mixer after preparation of a batch of cattle feed with monensin, lead to contamination of horse feed that was prepared immediately afterward in the same mixer. Six horses died as a result. (see "Ionophores" by Fritz and Hall in this issue of Veterinary Clinics of North America [VCNA]).

Horses are also extremely sensitive to the toxic effects of botulinum toxin produced by the bacterium, *Clostridium botulinum*. Under appropriate anaerobic conditions, these bacteria can grow in hay and produce botulinum toxin. When ingested as hay or hay products, serious, often fatal botulism can occur in horses or other livestock.[4]

In late 2022, a batch of alfalfa cubes was prepared using alfalfa that was contaminated with botulinum toxin. These were distributed in 10 states. In May 2023, it was reported that 98 horses were known to have been affected. Of these, at least 52 died or were euthanized. Since people can also be affected by botulinum toxin, warnings were sent out advising people to take caution when handling and disposing of the contaminated alfalfa cubes.[5]

Other feed recalls have been associated with detection of aflatoxin exceeding federal action levels, or misformulation resulting in excess concentrations of copper or selenium in the feed. Representative feed recalls are listed as follows.[6]

Horse Feed Recalls

2008 Aflatoxin—Horse feed recalled for aflatoxin exceeding FDA action levels. Distributed in 17 states.

2012 Monensin—Horse feed recalled. Distributed in NE and WY.

2014 Monensin—Horse feed recalled. Distributed in NC.

2015 Monensin—Horse feed recalled. Distributed in AZ and CA.

2015 Monensin—Horse feed delivered to one farm in FL.

2015 Copper—Livestock (including horses) feed recalled for excessive levels of copper.

2018 Monensin—Horse feed delivered to one farm in MN.

2019 Aflatoxin—Horse recalled. Distributed in GA, MD, NJ, NY, NC, PA, SC, VA, and WV.

2022 Botulinum toxin—Alfalfa Cubes recalled. Distributed in AR, CO, IL, KS, LA, MO, NM, OK, TX, and WI. Horse deaths in CO, LA, NM, and TX. Warnings for people to take caution when handling and disposing of the alfalfa cubes.

2023 Selenium—Horse feed recalled for elevated levels of selenium. Distributed in ID, MT, OR, and WA.

A list of feed product recalls and withdrawals is provided by the FDA at: https://www.fda.gov/animal-veterinary/safety-health/recalls-withdrawals.

SUMMARY

Given the enormous quantities of animal foods manufactured and sold, animal food products are generally safe and incidents of contamination are rare. Unfortunately, there are still cases in which feed–borne illness occurs in horses. The veterinarian plays a crucial role in recognizing these adverse events and in assessing the severity of animal and human health risk. Due to the possible severity and consequences of these outbreaks, proper reporting and consultation with government and state agencies are crucial. In these outbreaks, thorough case histories, and appropriate diagnostic testing allow accurate diagnoses, identification of the cause and elimination of the source through investigation and product recall.

CLINICS CARE POINTS

- Poisonings can present with a wide variety of clinical signs.
- In many instances, suspicion of poisoning can be related to a recent change in feed, or feeding from a new lot of feed, followed by the appearance of adverse clinical signs shortly thereafter, for example, in hours to days.
- Less commonly, suspicion of feed-related poisoning can occur when animals present with gradual loss of weight and condition during an extended period, for example, from weeks to months.
- After the case history is thoroughly documented, establishing differential diagnoses often begin with a complete necropsy and diagnostic testing.
- If there is any suspicion that a horse has died following ingestion of a toxic chemical, the carcass should never be sent for rendering.
- If there is heightened suspicion that a contaminant in the feed is the source of illness, then the veterinarian should report an animal food complaint to the FDA CVM.

ACKNOWLEDGMENTS

The author would like to gratefully acknowledge the contributions of Dr Christina R. Wilson-Frank to previous Veterinary Clinics of North America articles on Investigative Diagnostic Toxicology, parts of which are used in this article. Also gratefully acknowledged for assistance with article preparation is Conrad R. N. Hooser, A.S., Professional and Technical Writing.

DISCLOSURE

The author has neither commercial or financial conflicts of interest nor any funding sources to disclose. However, if you are aware of any potential funding sources (legal and legitimate only), please contact Dr S.B. Hooser at the address above.

REFERENCES

1. Jones J, Rottstein D, Ceric O, et al. Information for veterinarians on reporting suspected animal food issues. J Am Vet Med Assoc 2018;253:550–3.

2. Association of American Feed Control Officials (AAFCO). File a Complaint. Available at https://www.aafco.org/consumers/file-a-complaint/. Accessed October 25, 2023.

3. U.S. Food and Drug Administration. Reporting Problems with Horse or other Livestock Feed/Food. Content current as of 04/04/2023. Available at https://www.fda.gov/animal-veterinary/report-problem/reporting-problems-horse-or-other-livestock-feedfood. Accessed October 25, 2023.

4. Bischoff K, Moiseff J. Equine feed contamination and toxicology. Transl An Sci 2018;2:111–8.

5. U.S. Food and Drug Administration FDA Cautions horse owners not to feed recalled lots of Top of the Rockies Alfalfa Cubes due to reports of illness and death. Current as or 06/06/2023. https://www.fda.gov/animal-veterinary/outbreaks-and-advisories/fda-cautions-horse-owners-not-feed-recalled-lots-top-rockies-alfalfa-cubes-due-reports-illness-and Accessed October 25, 2023.

6. U.S. Food and Drug Administration. Guidance for Industry: Action Levels for Poisonous or Deleterious Substances in Human Food and Animal Feed. Content current as of 09/20/2018. Available at https://www.fda.gov/regulatory-information/search-fda-guidance-documents/guidance-industry-action-levels-poisonous-or-deleterious-substances-human-food-and-animal-feed. Accessed October 25, 2023.

Diagnostic Pathology of Equine Toxicoses

Lynne Cassone, DVM

KEYWORDS

- Equine • Pathology • Toxicosis • Necropsy • Diagnostic samples

KEY POINTS

- Observation of certain types and distributions of gross pathologic lesions during a complete pre- and/or postmortem examination may raise the index of suspicion for intoxication.
- Complete history, signalment, summary of gross findings, and photographs are essential for directing diagnostic efforts.
- Collection of appropriate specimens in adequate quantities will significantly increase the likelihood of a specific diagnosis.

INTRODUCTION

In general, toxicosis is a relatively rare cause of disease and death in horses, though it is often foremost in the client's mind when their horse suddenly (or not so suddenly) becomes ill, develops obvious external lesions, or dies. When the history includes a recent change in environment, feed, or management and multiple animals are reportedly affected in a short time frame, evaluation for a potential intoxication is definitely warranted.

Other chapters in this issue will be dedicated to in-depth study of potential toxicities in horses. This article is intended to highlight toxicosis-associated pathology that might be observed by a clinician in the living animal and at gross necropsy. Examples of toxicants that may cause the observed lesions are provided in this article, but these lists are not meant to be comprehensive. Although many toxicants can cause sudden death without observable clinical signs or gross pathology and there are very few pathognomonic gross lesions for a specific intoxicant, there are several peri- and postmortem changes that should raise the index of suspicion of intoxication. When the clinician is aware of these changes (particularly when coupled with a suggestive environmental or herd history), then collaboration with a diagnostic laboratory can begin to help identify specific toxicants. Proper sampling and communication with the diagnostic

Veterinary Diagnostic Laboratory, University of Kentucky, 1490 Bull Lea Road, Lexington, KY 40511, USA
E-mail address: Lynne.Cassone@uky.edu

Vet Clin Equine 40 (2024) 11–27
https://doi.org/10.1016/j.cveq.2023.10.005

laboratory will vastly improve the likelihood of a specific diagnosis; postmortem sampling and specimen submission are reviewed in the last section of this article.

EXTERNAL EXAMINATION

The obvious starting point for an external examination is the skin. Changes in skin may not necessarily be directly associated with fatal intoxication, but they occasionally occur in concert with systemic disease, and may point to a significant, potentially fatal systemic illness. In cases of toxicosis exclusively affecting skin, the disease may eventually progress to the point at which euthanasia is the only humane option; these intoxications are effectively, if not directly, fatal.

Grossly evident changes in skin include poor-quality hair coat, seborrhea, hypotrichosis/alopecia, edema, serous crusting, erosion/ulceration, and necrosis. Paying particular attention to the distribution of lesions (and noting this on a submission form, if biopsies are submitted) can be highly informative (**Table 1**).

Chronic selenosis is a classic example of a toxicant that can cause a generalized distribution of skin lesions, typically due to prolonged but sublethal consumption of selenium-accumulating plants or over-supplementation; changes include rough hair coat, alopecia, and irregular hoof growth or hoof sloughing. Chronic arsenic intoxication may have similar changes in a widespread distribution,[1,2] whereas the distribution of lesions associated with primary photosensitizing agents (eg, wild parsnip)[3] is limited to thinly haired and lightly pigmented skin; these toxins directly cause skin damage with ultraviolet light exposure, potentially causing hyperemia, epidermal necrosis, and scaling. Secondary hepatogenous photosensitizing agents elicit similar cutaneous lesions via hepatic metabolites. Pyrrolizidine alkaloids are the most commonly implicated plant-origin toxins that cause hepatogenous photosensitization.[4]

Depilatory agents (eg, mimosine, from *Mimosa pudica*)[5] and other toxins (eg, selenium, chronic arsenic)[2] that cause disruption of the hair cycle are most evident as

Table 1
Type and distribution of cutaneous lesions and some commonly associated toxicoses

Lesions	Examples
Mane and tail hair loss	Chronic selenosis, mimosine (*M pudica*)[1]
Coronary band, scaling, edema, crusting	Hepatotoxins (hepatocutaneous syndrome), Primary and hepatic photosensitization
Hoof wall, poor quality, sloughing	Chronic selenosis
Laminitis	Hoary alyssum (*Berteroa incana*); black walnut (*Juglans nigra*)
Generalized alopecia	Selenosis, arsenic
Generalized seborrhea	Arsenic, iodine toxicosis
Generalized necrosis	Primary photosensitization, arsenic
Generalized/ventral edema	Cardiotoxins (eg, ionophores)
Sparsely haired, and/or lightly or un-pigmented skin necrosis	Primary or hepatogenous photosensitization, acute arsenic
Extremities (head, neck limbs) with edema, necrosis	Snakebite
Limb edema	Hoary alyssum, black walnut
Limb necrosis	Ergotism
Urine scalding	Sorghum toxicosis

mane and tail hair loss, as these hairs grow continuously. The rest of the hair coat undergoes limited periods of seasonal growth and loss; alopecia may not be evident until failure to regrow hair after shedding is observed. Toxins which cause mane and tail hair loss also tend to cause hoof wall abnormalities, as this structure similarly grows continuously.

The coronary band (coronet) is a highly sensitive and dynamic cutaneous structure that is particularly susceptible to several toxicoses. Hepatocutaneous syndrome (aka, superficial necrolytic dermatitis) is a necrotizing and proliferative dermatosis associated with severe liver disease, including hepatotoxicosis, which may only manifest in this site.[6,7] This thinly haired area also may be the first or only site with evidence of photosensitization. Selenosis and ergotism may cause coronary band scaling, crusting, and edema, but lesions tend to be more widespread.[1,8]

Acute laminitis most likely will be diagnosed based on the horse's gait and stance, rather than an external examination; postmortem examination of sagittal sections of the hoof may reveal significant hyperemia and edema of laminae, but fortunately, most cases will not warrant euthanasia. Black walnut exposure is the most well-known toxicant that can cause laminar ischemia and pain; changes are typically reversible on the removal of black walnut shavings from the horse's environment.[9] Hoary alyssum, in contrast, may cause more severe, irreversible laminar disease.[10]

Unusual patterns of alopecia, seborrhea, or necrosis (eg, areas covered by blankets, tack, spray patterns, or sites of previous injury, and swelling) may be caused by exposure to a contact irritant or caustic chemical. Clients will occasionally "therapeutically" apply an astonishing array of caustic chemicals to skin (eg, bleach, lye, and creosote) and may not readily volunteer this information.

Non-cutaneous, external sites to examine include nasal and oral cavities, eyes, and perineum and external genitalia (**Table 2**). Effusions from various orifices can be highly informative. Copious nasal frothy fluid raises suspicion for cardiogenic pulmonary edema and heart failure, potentially associated with cardiotoxicosis (eg, ionophores).[11] A constellation of effusions, salivation, lacrimation, urination, diarrhea,

Table 2	
General external examination: non-cutaneous sites	
Lesions	**Examples**
Icterus of sclera and mucous membranes	Hepatotoxins (eg, alsike clover), hemolytic toxins (eg, maple)
Third eyelid prolapse	Tetanus, botulism
Nasal effusion, for example, foam/fluid/blood	Cardiotoxins (eg, *Taxus*)
Perineal fecal or blood-staining	Enteric toxicants (eg, NSAIDs)
Mucous membrane ulcerations	Blister beetles
Excessive salivation, lacrimation, sweating	Muscarinic signs (carbamates, organophosphates)
Feed accumulation in oropharynx	Delayed organophosphate, lead
Teeth: enamel hypoplasia, breakage, discoloration	Fluorosis
Bone: palpable irregular periosteal thickening	Vitamin D (eg, cholecalciferol rodenticides, over-supplementation)
Bone: increased fragility, pathologic fractures	Pulmonary silicosis
Muscle atrophy (neurogenic)	Delayed organophosphate, lead
Eyes: corneal edema, conjunctivitis	Photosensitization
Eyes: bilateral miosis	Organophosphates

and sweating, should evoke the vet school mnemonics of muscarinic agonist neuro-toxins (eg, acute exposure to carbamates, organophosphates). Excessive lacrimation associated with corneal edema and nonpurulent (initially) conjunctivitis may be early signs of photosensitization.[3]

Perineal staining with feces or melena indicates severe enteropathy. Although clearly infectious disease would be more likely in most cases, toxicosis targeting the intestinal mucosa is a reasonable and often overlooked differential; the presence of frank blood may be more suggestive of a toxic entity.

Clinically apparent neurogenic muscle atrophy may be caused by delayed neurotox-icosis and has been described as a specific delayed-onset syndrome of organophos-phate toxicosis due to neuronal "die-back."[12] Laryngeal and pharyngeal paralysis may be evident as dysphagia with accumulation of feed material in the mouth and increased salivation and are also potential outcomes of this toxicosis in horses.[13] Other causes of paresis of oropharynx and larynx include botulism, ergotism, and lead toxicosis.[8,14,15]

Teeth may exhibit brown discoloration and may be chalky or brittle, if the horse was exposed to excessive fluorine during tooth development. Fluorosis also may cause periosteal hyperostosis of the mandible and at tendinous or ligamentous insertions of long bones that may be palpable.[15] Hyperextended joints of the limbs and patho-logic fractures are reported with vitamin A toxicosis.[15]

Aborted or stillborn fetuses may exhibit skeletal deformities (locoweed/ *Astragalus*, *Oxytropis*), or ankyloses/arthrogryposis (hybrid sorghum, Sudan grass).[16,17] Observa-tions compatible with ergovaline (toxic endophyte-infected tall fescue) toxicosis or ergotism include premature placental separation ("red bag"), advanced gestational age, and agalactia.[8] Newborn foals with enlarged thyroids may have been exposed to excessive iodine during development.[15]

INTERNAL EXAMINATION

In the unfortunate circumstance that the patient does not survive or when the only clin-ical sign is sudden death, a complete postmortem examination is the logical next step in the diagnostic workup. For a handy, concise, instructional manual on performing a complete gross examination, tissue sampling, and differentiation of lesions from arti-facts, there is no better reference than The Necropsy Book, currently in its 7th edi-tion.[18] All organs have a limited range of grossly visible changes in response to injury, regardless of whether the etiology is infectious/inflammatory, degenerative, toxic, and so forth. Differentiation between infectious and noninfectious disease is oc-casionally possible with gross examination alone, though there is often significant overlap in the appearance of gross lesions of acute inflammatory and toxic diseases. As with lesions in the skin, identification of the distribution of lesions is a key: systemic toxicoses are nearly always symmetric and evenly distributed throughout an anatomic structure.

At the bare minimum, both pleural and peritoneal spaces should be opened. In cases with neurologic symptoms or unwitnessed or sudden death, brain also should be removed and examined. Ideally, brain would be examined and sampled in every case, though the reality is that most clinicians find brain removal in the field too daunting.

Pathologic changes should be carefully noted in a gross description that should accompany specimens sent to a diagnostic laboratory for further testing. Although there are toxins that cause specific lesions that are virtually pathognomonic, these are often reported more frequently than their actual incidence would warrant (because they are so very photogenic).

Internal Viscera on Whole

Generalized edema, petechiation, ecchymoses, and organ congestion are common in sudden death caused by a number of etiologies, including infectious and toxic diseases. These changes are usually the end result of an irreversible imbalance of inflammatory cytokines, vasoactive substances, and/or disruption of the balance of coagulation/fibrinolysis (eg, disseminated intravascular coagulopathy). Toxins which target oxidative phosphorylation functions of the mitochondria, such as aluminum phosphide and cyanide,[19,20] will directly cause these widespread changes due to rapid depletion of energy and subsequent cell death of all tissues. Anticoagulant rodenticide intoxication also may cause widespread hemorrhages in all tissues, with or without significant cavitary bleeding; hemorrhage of the diaphragmatic aponeurosis is a common finding in cases of systemic hemorrhage or blood loss of any etiology (**Fig. 1**).[21,22]

Generalized discoloration of viscera and soft tissues may be striking. Brown discoloration is compatible with methemoglobinemia (eg, red maple/*Acer rubrum*; **Fig. 2**),[23] whereas generalized icterus may be due to severe bile stasis (eg, the aptly named toxin, icterogenin of the ornamental shrub, *Lantana camara*)[24] or hemolysis.

Enzootic calcinosis caused by calcitriol-containing plants (eg, *Cestrum diurnum*) and metastatic mineralization (vitamin D over-supplementation, cholecalciferol rodenticide, renal failure) may affect multiple sites and may be obvious on first opening the body. The walls of large-caliber arteries will be firm, non-pliable, and possibly gritty. Lungs may not fully collapse due to alveolar mineralization. Pleural surfaces may contain white flecks or plaques ("pleural frosting"). Other potential sites of mineral deposition include kidney, heart (myocardium and endocardium), muscle, ligaments and tendons.[25,26]

Body Cavities

Transudate, modified transudate, and frank blood are effusions into the pleural, peritoneal, and/or pericardial spaces that may be associated with a toxicosis. Transudates and modified transudates may be observed with generalized edema (see above), and heart failure (see below). Frank blood with or without apparent coagulation may be caused by anticoagulant rodenticide poisoning or consumption of moldy sweet clover (*Melilotus* sp).[8]

Blood

Changes in color and consistency of blood are generally not subtle and can be extremely useful in identifying potential toxic etiologies. Brown discoloration is compatible with methemoglobinemia, which is highly suggestive of red maple (*A rubrum*) or *Pistacia* toxicosis.[23] Bright red venous blood occurs when oxygen is not effectively utilized by cells, which may be an indication of a toxin that targets oxidative phosphorylation (eg, phosphine, peracute cyanide); if animals survive for 30 to 60 minutes, the blood will eventually turn dark red and will not clot.[19,20,27] The failure of blood to coagulate may indicate anticoagulant rodenticide or moldy sweet clover (*Melilotus* sp) intoxication.[8,21,22]

Skeletal Muscle

Skeletal musculature comprises around half of a horse's total body weight. Although limited areas of myonecrosis/rhabdomyolysis (eg, localized infection, trauma) may not have significant systemic effects, toxic myopathy is often widespread and may cause severe myoglobinuria resulting in renal failure or respiratory failure by damaging muscles of the diaphragm. Owing to the sheer mass of tissue involved, widespread

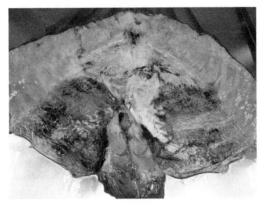

Fig. 1. Diaphragmatic hemorrhage, anticoagulant rodenticide intoxication.

necrosis may also induce overwhelming inflammatory cytokines and other pro-inflammatory mediators that precipitate cardiovascular collapse.

Primary gross changes that may be observed include hemorrhage, edema, necrosis, and mineralization. Necrosis may appear as patchy areas of severe pallor and/or dark red discoloration. Examples of toxins that can directly damage skeletal muscle include ionophores,[11] organophosphates,[12] cantharidin,[28] and numerous plants, including box elder (*Acer negundo*; seasonal pasture myopathy),[29] *Senna spp.* plants, and white snakeroot (*Eupatorium rugosum*).[30]

Bone

The most easily examined bones on internal examination are the ribs, though distal long bones also can be easily exposed, and flat bones of the skull during brain removal. Similar to other organs, bilateral symmetry and involvement of multiple sites are flags that a systemic toxicosis is a possible cause of bone disease. Bones may exhibit altered thickness (periosteal hyperostosis), irregular or roughened periosteal and articular surfaces, osteoporosis/fragility and pathologic fractures, and osteodystrophy (**Fig. 3**). The latter can be examined by cutting longitudinally through a physis, revealing one or more bands of aberrant sclerosis in the distal metaphysis caused by impaired

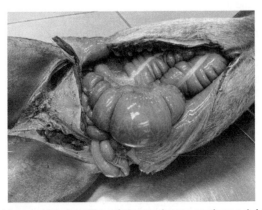

Fig. 2. Generalized brown discoloration of tissues due to methemoglobinemia, red maple toxicosis. (*Courtesy of* L. Kennedy, DVM DACVP.)

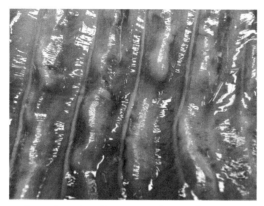

Fig. 3. Ribs from an aborted equine fetus seventh month gestation; possible teratogen exposure.

osteoclastic resorption; lead intoxication may be characterized by multiple lines of sclerosis,[16] while vitamin D typically manifests as a single line, which may be preceded by an area of rarefaction (**Fig. 4**). Other potential toxicities of bone include fluorosis,[31] lead,[15] and equine bone fragility syndrome caused by pulmonary silicosis.[32]

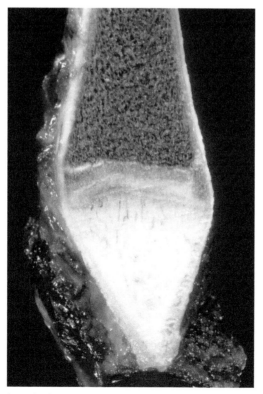

Fig. 4. Distal metaphyseal sclerosis, vitamin D toxicosis. (*Courtesy of* John F Edwards, DVM, PhD, DACVP.)

Brain

Some toxicants cause specific and easily detected microscopic lesions in brain, while grossly the range of tissue reaction is more limited and nonspecific compared to other organs - congestion, edema (which may manifest as flattened gyri or coning of the cerebellum), and severe malacia. Exceptions include fumonisins, which can cause a particularly striking and widespread leukoencephalomalacia,[8] and nigropalladial encephalomalacia, a highly targeted focus of necrosis of the substantia nigra and globus pallidus that is pathognomonic for *Centaurea* spp. (eg, yellow star thistle) toxicosis; it is worth noting that in violation of the general principle more or less bilateral symmetry of lesions of toxicoses, this lesion may be unilateral.[33–35]

Oro/nasopharynx

Severe congestion and/or edema of the nasal and pharyngeal mucosa, and possibly presence of impacted feed material may point to pharyngeal paresis or paralysis, compatible with botulism,[14] fumonisins,[8] lead,[15] chronic organophosphate,[13] or other neurodegenerative or paralytic toxins.[33–35]

Trachea and Lungs

Severe edema and large quantities of clear, colorless, or red-tinged foamy fluid filling the trachea and large airways may be seen with acute heart failure, direct damage to alveolar capillaries or respiratory epithelium, and pathologic increase in secretions (muscarinic effect). Ionophore toxicosis is a relatively common cause of acute myocardial toxicosis in horses, usually due to accidental ingestion of medicated feed intended for cattle or chickens,[11] and often presents as fatal pulmonary edema. Yew (*Taxus spp.*)[36] and *oleander*[37] similarly may cause peracute cardiogenic edema.[36,37] The direct damage to pulmonary tissues is less common and may be caused by ketones of perilla mint,[38] oxygen toxicity, or pyrrolizidine alkaloids.[39] Differentiation of this pattern of lung damage from a primary inflammatory disease (eg, viral infection or acute respiratory disease syndrome) can be challenging, even on histologic examination.[40] Documentation of possible exposure to toxicants or acute onset of disease in multiple animals may help make this determination.

Although pulmonary consolidation is much more commonly the result of infectious/inflammatory disease, the herbicide paraquat[41] and Crofton weed (sticky snakeroot; *Ageratina adenophora*)[42] may cause similar gross changes in the lungs which will appear diffusely firm. Subacute or chronic stages of pulmonary injury caused by pulmonary toxicants described above also can cause proliferative and/or sclerosing pneumonitis and grossly apparent pulmonary consolidation.[39,40]

Lungs with widely disseminated, small, gritty foci may have pulmonary silicosis. Assessment for evidence of osteoporosis and bone fragility may be warranted.[32]

The failure of nonconsolidated lung parenchyma to collapse postmortem may indicate mineralization of alveolar walls (metastatic mineralization), which may be a primary lesion of vitamin D toxicosis[26] (**Fig. 5**) or secondary to renal failure (uremic pneumonitis).[15,39]

Cardiovascular

The heart is a common target of peracute fatal intoxications due to the susceptibility of the organ to electrolyte abnormalities, to even relatively minor lesions that may impact the conduction system and to acute myocardial ischemia and/or necrosis.

Because of the often limited clinical course of disease, clinical cardiac insufficiency or failure caused by intoxication often precedes development of grossly visible

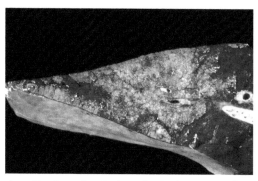

Fig. 5. Pulmonary mineralization, vitamin D toxicosis. (*Courtesy of* John F Edwards, DVM, PhD, DACVP.)

lesions, and even microscopic lesions in peracute cases can be equivocal. Gross lesions that may be observed include multifocal areas of pallor suggesting ischemic necrosis (white snakeroot/*Ageratina altissima,*[43] rayless goldenrod/*Isocoma pluriflora*[44]), congestion and hemorrhage (cantharidin,[28] ionophores,[11] *Taxus*[36]; **Fig. 6**), and mineralization (vitamin D and analogs[25,26]).[45] The large papillary muscles tend to be more susceptible to toxicologic and ischemic insult and are good sites to section submit for histopathology. Epicardial hemorrhage is common in peracute cardiotoxicity, and increased pericardial fluid, even without gross lesions of the myocardium itself, is often seen with microscopic evidence of acute myocardial damage.

Large-caliber arteries are frequent sites of intimal to transmural mineralization associated with metastatic mineralization (eg, enzootic calcinosis,[25] vitamin D toxicosis[15,26]). These will be obvious when dissecting out organs; they palpate very firm and gritty and may be difficult to cut (**Fig. 7**).

Liver

Given that liver is responsible for the detoxification of the majority of endogenous and exogenous toxins, it is also the most common target and mediator of toxicoses. Numerous chemical agents are directly hepatotoxic, whereas others are converted to their toxic principles by hepatic enzymes. Gross changes include yellow or tan discoloration due to necrosis, hydropic degeneration, or lipid accumulation; orange-brown discoloration due to bile stasis; friability due to dissociation of hepatocytes or hepatocellular necrosis; and diffuse fibrosis/cirrhosis. Occasionally no gross

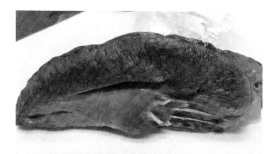

Fig. 6. Bovine heart with myocardial necrosis, ionophore intoxication.

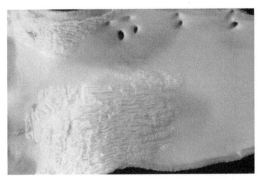

Fig. 7. Arterial intimal mineralization, vitamin D toxicosis. (*Courtesy of* John F Edwards, DVM, PhD, DACVP.)

changes are apparent, whereas histologically severe liver disease can be discerned. Common hepatotoxins of horses include microcystin (blue-green algae),[24] fumonisins, and other mycotoxins,[8] and pyrrolizidine alkaloids present in several plant species.[24]

Kidney and Urinary Bladder

Similar to liver, the proximal renal tubules are a common target for toxicologic agents due to their high metabolic activity coupled with near-continuous exposure to toxins and metabolites in the ultrafiltrate emanating from renal glomeruli. Dehydration and hypovolemia will significantly increase the likelihood of toxic damage to renal parenchyma due to increased concentration of toxins in the ultrafiltrate and decreased metabolic support of tubular epithelia.

Gross evidence of toxicosis in kidneys includes bilateral, diffuse discoloration (pale tan, yellow/icteric, or dark brown/black), congestion, friability, swelling, crystalluria, focal yellow–brown discoloration (necrosis) along the renal papillary crest (eg, NSAIDs), swelling, and edema.[46] Pelvic hemorrhage is occasionally seen with cantharidin/blister beetle toxicosis.[28] Kidneys and perirenal connective tissue may be severely edematous (acorn/tannins of *Quercus spp*).[47]

The urinary bladder mucosa may contain mucosal to transmural hemorrhages with cantharidin toxicosis[28] (**Fig. 8**). Urine may be discolored red–brown (hemoglobinuria, myoglobinuria, bilirubinuria).[23,46]

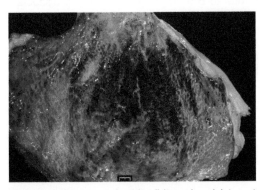

Fig. 8. Urinary bladder hemorrhage, cantharidin (blister beetle) intoxication. (*Courtesy of* John F Edwards, DVM, PhD, DACVP.)

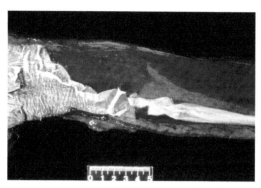

Fig. 9. Esophageal ulceration and hemorrhage, cantharidin (blister beetle) intoxication. (*Courtesy of* John F Edwards, DVM, PhD, DACVP.)

Esophagus and Gastrointestinal Tract

As the equine clinician well knows, the esophagus is a problematic segment of the alimentary canal in equids. Acute ulceration and necrosis may not be fatal, but scarring, stenosis, and choke are common sequelae. Multiple linear ulcerations of the esophageal mucosa are features of cantharidin[28] and arsenic intoxication[15,48,49] (**Fig. 9**). Acquired megaesophagus is a classic lesion of lead toxicosis in many species and has been observed in the horse (JF Edwards, personal communication, 2023).

The gastric glandular mucosa is likewise susceptible to ulceration and hemorrhage. Severe glandular mucosal hyperemia is common and may precede widespread mucosal hemorrhage; the very commonly observed ulceration of nonglandular mucosa along the margo plicatus is *not* generally associated with toxicosis. Arsenicals,[15,48] cantharidin,[28] and non-steroidal anti-inflammatory drugs (NSAIDs)[49] have frequently been implicated in these changes, as well as causing similar lesions in the intestinal tract; dorsal large colon is particularly susceptible (**Fig. 10**). The resulting toxic injury may present as hemorrhagic diarrhea, hematochezia, or melena. Additional potential toxic etiologies of gastrointestinal damage include paraquat,[41] lead,[15] and oleander.[37] Gastric mucosa is a common site for metastatic mineralization; gross lesions are typically subtle, white "frosting" of the mucosal surface. Vitamin D toxicosis and renal failure are potential causes.[26,46]

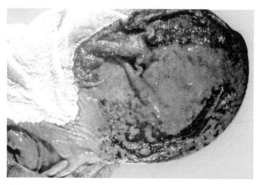

Fig. 10. Gastric glandular mucosal hemorrhage, arsenic intoxication. (*Courtesy of* John F Edwards, DVM, PhD, DACVP.)

Table 3
Internal examination gross changes and common toxin differentials

Lesions	Examples
Brain	
General meningeal congestion, edema, flattening of gyri, cerebellar coning	Lead, organomercurials, salt toxicosis
Cerebral cortex predominant malacia	Fumonisins
Brainstem/nigropallidal encephalomalacia: note that this lesion may be unilateral	*Centaurea* spp (eg, yellow starthistle)
Respiratory tract	
Nasal mucosa, pharynx, larynx, trachea: edema, congestion, presence of feed material	Pharyngeal/laryngeal paresis (eg, botulism, fumonisins, lead, delayed organophosphate)
Lung aspiration pneumonia	Pharyngeal paresis: see above
Pulmonary edema	Heart failure (eg, ionophores) Direct pulmonary toxicant (eg, perilla mint/*Perilla frutescens*, 3-methyl indole) Muscarinic-induced tracheobronchial secretion (eg, carbamates, organophosphates)
Pulmonary consolidation/fibrosis	Paraquat, Crofton weed/sticky snakeroot (*A adenophora*); chronic lung injury.
Cardiovascular system	
Pleural, peritoneal, and/or pericardial clear effusions	Heart failure (eg, oleander; *Nerium oleander*) Hypoproteinemia (eg, arsenic)
Heart: myocardial congestion/hemorrhage (dark red discoloration)	Blister beetles
Heart: necrosis (pallor, soft)	White snakeroot (*A altissima*)
Heart: mineralization	Vitamin D (eg, over-supplementation of vitamin D3)
Blood/viscera: brown: methemoglobinemia	Maples (eg, *A rubrum*) and pistachios
Blood: Bright red venous blood	Cyanide (eg, chokecherry; *Prunus virginiana*)
Blood/viscera: Bright pink	Carbon monoxide (eg, barn fire)
Alimentary tract	
Oral cavity (ulcers, food accumulation)	Pharyngeal paresis (eg, lead)
Tongue, esophagus, stomach, small intestine, and/or colon: ulcers, hemorrhage	Blister beetle, acorn
Diarrhea/watery intestinal contents	Arsenic, acorn
Small intestine, colon: ileus	Atropine
Hepatobiliary	
Liver: swelling, friability, discoloration (dark red/congestion, pallor/lipid)	Acute hepatotoxins (eg, blue–green algae microcystins)
Liver: small, firm, irregular surface (cirrhosis/fibrosis)	Chronic hepatotoxins (eg, pyrrolizidine alkaloid-containing plants)
Liver: cholestasis (yellow/brown discoloration)	Pyrrolizidine alkaloid-containing plants (eg, *Senecio* spp)

(continued on next page)

Table 3
(continued)

Lesions	Examples
Liver: prominent reticular pattern ("nutmeg" liver) chronic passive congestion, portal fibrosis	Subacute to subchronic hepatopathy or right-sided cardiac insufficiency
Urinary tract	
Kidneys: Red discoloration, diffuse or streaking	Blister beetle, aminoglycosides
Kidneys: Renal papillary necrosis (multifocal, yellow–brown discoloration)	NSAIDs
Urinary bladder: ulceration	Blister beetle
Urinary bladder: hemorrhage	Anticoagulant rodenticide
Urine: brown, red pigmenturia (bilirubinuria, hemoglobinuria, myoglobinuria)	Hepatoxicosis, hemolysis, rhabdomyolysis, (eg, box elder, *A negundo*)
Musculoskeletal and hooves	
Skeletal muscle: hemorrhage, edema, necrosis (pallor, and/or dark red discoloration)	Rhabdomyolysis (eg, box elder)
Skeletal muscle: mineralization	Vitamin D (eg, *C diurnum*)
Diaphragm: hemorrhage	Anticoagulants (eg, rodenticides)
Bone, joints, teeth: discoloration, degradation	Chronic fluorosis
Bone: osteodystrophy (radiographic "lead lines")	Lead, vitamin D
Hooves: sagittal sections: laminitis, coronary congestion/edema	Hoary alyssum

Horses with significant life-threatening secretory diarrhea may not have grossly obvious intestinal pathology aside from the profuse watery contents. For example, sulfur toxicosis in horses causes severe osmotic diarrhea, which may be sufficient to cause significant electrolyte abnormalities (horses do not develop thiamine deficiency and polioencephalomalacia, the hallmark disease of sulfur toxicosis in ruminants).[50] Acorn toxicosis may be associated with either severe intestinal edema and diarrhea or necrohemorrhagic colitis.[47]

Hooves

Sagittal sections of hooves may reveal acute laminitis changes (eg, laminar severe congestion and edema) that are not apparent radiographically. Toxins that routinely result in severe laminitis include black walnut and hoary alyssum.[9,10] **Table 3** lists the examples of gross pathologic changes and a few possible associated toxicologic etiologies.

SAMPLE COLLECTION

Matthews[51] refers to an unproven law that in this context predicts that the more certain the diagnostician is that no toxicant is involved, the more likely it will seem that intoxication has occurred. This probability increases in the direct proportion with the value of the horse and litigiousness of the owner and increases exponentially if inadequate samples for toxicologic testing are collected.

Table 4 Diagnostic samples: quantities		
Specimen	**Fresh/Frozen**	**Fixed**
Liver	20 g	3 sites
Kidney	20 g	2 sites, including cortex and medulla
Skeletal muscle	20 g	diaphragm, 1 other site
Brain	20 g (minimum) Hemisphere preferred	cortex, midbrain, brain stem, cerebellum
Heart	20 g	Right/left ventricular free walls septum
Spleen	NA	1 site
Stomach	1 cup contents	1 stomach wall (margo plicatus)
Small intestine		3 sites: duodenum, jejunum, ileum
Colon	1 cup contents	2 sites ventral, dorsal large colon
Feces	1 cup	NA
Urine	10 mL	1 site urinary bladder
Fat	20 g	NA
Eye fluid	aqueous, vitreous 1 mL/each ideal	NA
Whole blood	10 mL red top 5 mL purple top*	NA
Cerebrospinal fluid	10 mL	NA
Feeds and supplements	Include labels or photos of labels Entire bags preferred; 1 gallon bag minimum	NA
Forages	Multiple flakes of square bales Any grossly affected areas; unusual plants, and so forth	NA
Suspect plants	Entire plant if possible, can also include photos of large plants (eg, trees)	NA

Therefore, it behooves the diagnostician to routinely collect adequate and appropriate samples for toxicologic testing. When multiple animals are affected, this becomes imperative.

A complete necropsy gives the diagnostician the opportunity to collect a wide array of specimens appropriate for attaining a diagnosis, toxicologic, or otherwise. Sample containers and temporary storage are relatively inexpensive compared with the frustration of failing to make a diagnosis due to the lack of appropriate specimens.

Table 4 provides a comprehensive list of samples to collect. In cases in which toxicosis is under strong suspicion (eg, sudden death with no premonitory signs, multiple animals affected, recent changes in environment, and feed), collection of all samples drastically increases the likelihood of a specific diagnosis.

In addition to the samples listed, if hemolysis and anemia are significant clinical findings, inclusion of blood for complete blood count, a blood smear, and bone marrow (roll preparation for cytology, and fixed) may aid in diagnosis of intoxication or other possible primary diseases of blood and bone marrow (immune-mediated, infectious, neoplastic).

Fixed specimens can be pooled in one container. Adequate fixation requires sections 5 mm thick or less and a minimum of 1:10 ratio of tissue volume to neutral buffered formalin; that is, fresh tissue should occupy no more than 1/10th of the container volume.[18] To simplify shipping, fixed tissue may be held overnight in the 1:10 volume of formalin and then transferred to a much smaller volume (just enough to cover tissues) for shipment; be sure to note that the specimens were fixed in 1:10 formalin before packaging for shipping to avoid receiving "educational material" on proper fixation volumes from the receiving laboratory's quality control department.

Although the preceding provides a general approach to field necropsy sample collection, consultation with a diagnostic laboratory is the best way to ensure that the most appropriate specimens are collected and for advice regarding technique (eg, brain removal, fixation, and shipping), and diagnostic laboratory professionals may propose possible differentials based on the observed clinical signs and lesions. Diagnosticians live for this. So, please call.

CLINICS CARE POINTS

- Careful documentation of history is essential. Herd health and environmental changes may point toward possible toxicosis. Multiple animals affected in a relatively short timeframe, and recent changes in pasture, feed, water, and so forth are examples of possible flags.

- Notation of distribution of lesions can be highly informative, with few exceptions, approximately bilateral symmetry and tracking of lesions along specific anatomic structures (eg, diffusely accentuated hepatic lobular pattern, or necrosis specifically of lightly pigmented skin), are more likely to be due to metabolic/toxic disease.

- complete postmortem examination and an appropriate sampling of tissues from all body cavities and brain vastly increase the likelihood of a specific diagnosis.

- If the case is not routine (and most toxicologic cases are not), personal communication with your diagnostic laboratory is strongly encouraged before submitting samples.

DISCLOSURE

None.

REFERENCES

1. Scott DW, Miller WH. Equine dermatology-E-book, Chemical toxicoses. Elsevier Health Sciences; 2011. p. 408–9.
2. Maxie G. Jubb, Kennedy & Palmer's pathology of domestic animals, Volume 1: Chemical injury to skin. Elsevier health sciences, 2015. pp 566-572.
3. Winter JC, Thieme K, Eule JC, et al. Photodermatitis and ocular changes in nine horses after ingestion of wild parsnip (pastinaca sativa). BMC Vet Res 2022; 18(1):80.
4. Scott DW, Miller WH. Equine dermatology-E-book, Photosensitization. Elsevier Health Sciences; 2011. p. pp413–7.
5. Scott DW, Miller WH. Equine dermatology, plant toxicoses. Elsevier Health Sciences; 2011. p. pp410–1.
6. Scott DW, Miller WH. Equine dermatology, Coronary Band Disorders. Elsevier Health Sciences; 2011. p. pp462–3.
7. Maxie G. Jubb, Kennedy & Palmer's pathology of domestic animals, Volume 1: superficial necrolytic dermatitis. Elsevier health sciences; 2015. p. 586–7.

8. Hintz H. Molds, mycotoxins, and mycotoxicosis. Vet Clin N Am Equine Pract 1990;6(2):419–31.

9. Adair H, Goble DO, Schmidhammer JL, et al. Laminar microvascular flow, measured by means of laser Doppler flowmetry, during the prodromal stages of black walnut-induced laminitis in horses. Am J Vet Res 2000;61:862–8.

10. Geor R, Becker R, Kanara E, et al. Toxicosis in horses after ingestion of hoary alyssum. J Am Vet Med Assoc 1992;201(1):63–7.

11. Blomme E, La Perle KM, Wilkins PA, et al. Ionophore toxicity in horses. Equine Vet Educ 1999;11(3):153–8.

12. Myers C, Aleman M, Heidmann P, et al. Myopathy in American miniature horses. Equine Vet J 2006;38(3):272–6.

13. Duncan I, Brook D. Bilateral laryngeal paralysis in the horse. Equine Vet J 1985; 17(3):228–33.

14. Galey FD. Botulism in the horse. Vet Clin N Am Equine Pract 2001;17(3):579–88.

15. Schryver H. Mineral and vitamin intoxication in horses. Vet Clin N Am Equine Pract 1990;6(2):295–318.

16. Maxie G. Jubb, Kennedy & Palmer's pathology of domestic animals, Volume 1: Toxic Bone Diseases Elsevier health sciences, 2015. pp 84-91.

17. Panter KE, Welch KD, Gardner DR, et al. Poisonous plants: effects on embryo and fetal development. Birth defects research Part C: Embryo today: reviews 2013;99(4):223–34.

18. King JM, Roth-Johnson L, Dodd DC, et al. The Necropsy Book: a guide for veterinary students, residents, clinicians, pathologists, and biological researchers. The Internet-First University Press; 2014.

19. Easterwood L, Chaffin MK, Marsh PS, et al. Phosphine intoxication following oral exposure of horses to aluminum phosphide–treated feed. J Am Vet Med Assoc 2010;236(4):446–50.

20. Mosing M, Kuemmerle JM, Dadak A, et al. Metabolic changes associated with anaesthesia and cherry poisoning in a pony. Vet Anaesth Analg 2009;36(3):255–60.

21. Ayala I, Rodríguez MJ, Martos N, et al. Fatal brodifacoum poisoning in a pony. Can Vet J 2007;48(6):627.

22. Carvallo FR, Poppenga R, Kinde H, et al. Cluster of cases of massive hemorrhage associated with anticoagulant detection in race horses. J Vet Diagn Invest 2015; 27(1):112–6.

23. Alward A, Corriher CA, Barton MH, et al. Red maple (Acer rubrum) leaf toxicosis in horses: a retrospective study of 32 cases. J Vet Intern Med 2006;20(5):1197–201.

24. Maxie G. Jubb, Kennedy & Palmer's pathology of domestic animals: Vol 2, liver and biliary system. Elsevier health sciences; 2015. p. 293.

25. Krook L, Wasserman R, Shively J, et al. Hypercalcemia and calcinosis in Florida horses: implication of the shrub, Cestrum diurnum, as the causative agent. Cornell Vet 1975;65(1):26–56.

26. Harrington D, Page E. Acute vitamin D3 toxicosis in horses: case reports and experimental studies of the comparative toxicity of vitamins D2 and D3. J Am Vet Med Assoc 1983;182(12):1358–69.

27. Maxie G. Jubb, Kennedy & Palmer's pathology of domestic animals: Vol 1, anoxia and anoxic poisons. Elsevier health sciences; 2015. p. 305.

28. Schmitz D. Cantharidin toxicosis in horses. J Vet Intern Med 1989;3(4):208–15.

29. Valberg SJ, Sponseller B, Hegeman AD, et al. Seasonal pasture myopathy/atypical myopathy in North A merica associated with ingestion of hypoglycin A within seeds of the box elder tree. Equine Vet J 2013;45(4):419–26.

30. Maxie G. Jubb, Kennedy & Palmer's pathology of domestic animals: Vol 1, Toxic myopathies. Elsevier health sciences; 2015. p. 218–9.
31. Kelly LH, Uzal FA, Poppenga RH, et al. Equine dental and skeletal fluorosis induced by well water consumption. J Vet Diagn Invest 2020;32(6):942–7.
32. Arens A, Barr B, Puchalski S, et al. Osteoporosis associated with pulmonary silicosis in an equine bone fragility syndrome. Veterinary pathology 2011;48(3): 593–615.
33. Cordy D. Nigropallidal encephalomalacia in horses associated with ingestion of yellow star thistle. J Neuropathol Exp Neurol 1954;13:330–42.
34. Ruby RE, Janes JG. Pathologic Conditions of the Nervous System in Horses. Vet Clin Equine Pract 2022;38(2):427–43.
35. Maxie G. Jubb, Kennedy & Palmer's pathology of domestic animals, Volume 1: Neurodegenerative diseases. Elsevier health sciences, 2015, p317.
36. Tiwary AK, Puschner B, Kinde H, et al. Diagnosis of Taxus (yew) poisoning in a horse. J Vet Diagn Invest 2005;17(3):252–5.
37. Galey FD, Holstege DM, Plumlee KH, et al. Diagnosis of oleander poisoning in livestock. J Vet Diagn Invest 1996 Jul;8(3):358–64.
38. Breeze R, Laegreid W, Bayly W, et al. Perilla ketone toxicity: a chemical model for the study of equine restrictive lung disease. Equine Vet J 1984;16(3):180–4.
39. Maxie G. Jubb, Kennedy & Palmer's pathology of domestic animals, Volume 2: Toxic lung injury. Elsevier health sciences, 2015, pp518-519.
40. Buergelt C, Hines S, Cantor G, et al. A retrospective study of proliferative interstitial lung disease of horses in Florida. Veterinary Pathology 1986;23(6):750–6.
41. Nagy A, Cortinovis C, Spicer L, et al. Long-established and emerging pesticide poisoning in horses. Equine Vet Educ 2019;31(9):496–500.
42. Shapter FM, Granados-Soler JL, Stewart AJ, et al. Equine Crofton Weed (Ageratina spp.) Pneumotoxicity: What Do We Know and What Do We Need to Know? Animals 2023;13(13):2082.
43. Smetzer D, Coppock R, Ely R, et al. Cardiac effects of white snakeroot intoxication in horses. Equine Pract 1983;5(2):26–32.
44. Davis T, Stegelmeier B, Lee S, et al. Experimental rayless goldenrod (Isocoma pluriflora) toxicosis in horses. Toxicon 2013;73:88–95.
45. Maxie G. Jubb, Kennedy & Palmer's pathology of domestic animals, Volume 3: Myocardial disease. Elsevier health sciences, 2015, pp34-38.
46. Maxie G. Jubb, Kennedy & Palmer's pathology of domestic animals, Volume 2: Acute tubular injury. Elsevier health sciences, 2015, pp424-427.
47. Smith S, Naylor R, Knowles E, et al. Suspected acorn toxicity in nine horses. Equine Vet J 2015;47(5):568–72.
48. Pace L, Turnquist S, Casteel S, et al. Acute arsenic toxicosis in five horses. Veterinary pathology 1997;34(2):160–4.
49. Maxie G. Jubb, Kennedy & Palmer's pathology of domestic animals, Volume 2: Stomach. Elsevier health sciences, 2015, pp51-55.
50. Burgess BA, Lohmann KL, Blakley BR. Excessive sulfate and poor water quality as a cause of sudden deaths and an outbreak of diarrhea in horses. Can Vet J 2010;51(3):277.
51. Matthews RA. The science of Murphy's law. Paper presented at. Proceedings-royal institution of great Britain; 1999.

Plants

Range and Pasture Plants Likely to Poison Horses

Bryan L. Stegelmeier, DVM, PhD*, T. Zane Davis, PhD

KEYWORDS

- Range and pasture • Poisonous plants • Equine • Poisoning • Diagnosis
- Treatment

KEY POINTS

- Locoweed poisoning requires continuous long exposure to produce irreversible neurologic disease.
- Early spring growth of poison hemlock is eaten and can poison horses, but most recover from poisoning if they are allowed to calmly clear the toxin.
- Oxalate-containing plants generally cause chronic poisoning in horses that can result in nutritional hyperparathyroidism and fibrous osteodystrophy.
- Knapweed and yellow star thistle poison horses, mules, and donkeys producing nigropallidal encephalomalacia.
- Photosensitization in horses can be plant induced (primary photosensitization) or due to plant-induced hepatic failure and hepatogenic photosensitization.

Locoweed poisoning or "Locoism" in horses is a neurologic disease historically considered to be the largest poisonous plant problem in the western United States.[1,2] Locoweeds are indigenous plants with huge, long-lived seed banks such that herbicide and removal is short lived and temporary. Horses are uniquely susceptible to poisoning. Not only do horses require lower swainsonine doses to develop neurologic disease, but they also require relatively short exposure durations to develop irreversible neurologic impairment. Even more dangerous is that horses readily eat most locoweeds, irrespective of alternative forage availability.

Locoweeds include about 20 species of the *Astragalus* and *Oxytropis* genera that contain swainsonine (**Fig. 1**A–C). Swainsonine, an endophyte-produced indolizidine alkaloid, inhibits lysosomal α-mannosidase and mannosidase II.[3] This results in lysosomal accumulation of mannose-rich oligosaccharides. Microscopically this is seen as characteristic visceral and neuronal vacuolation. Within individually affected cells, lesions are biochemically, morphologically, and clinically indistinguishable from genetic mannosidosis.[4] Swainsonine, the endophytes that produce it, and similar induced

USDA/ARS Poisonous Plant Research Laboratory, 1150 East 1400 North, Logan, UT 84341, USA
* Corresponding author. 1150 East 1400 North, Logan, UT 84341.
E-mail address: Bryan.Stegelmeier@USDA.GOV

Vet Clin Equine 40 (2024) 29–44
https://doi.org/10.1016/j.cveq.2023.12.002
0749-0739/24/© 2024 Elsevier Inc. All rights reserved.
vetequine.theclinics.com

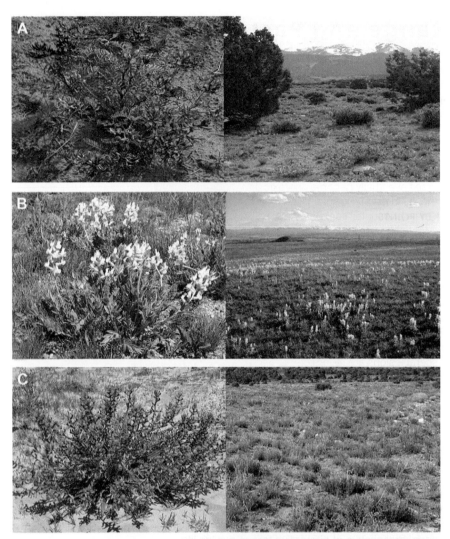

Fig. 1. Photographs of commonly locoweeds and the habitat in which they grow. These are the most common locoweeds that poison horses in North America—(A) *Astragalus lentiginosus* or spotted locoweed. This locoweed has over 50 location-dependent varieties. These are native perennial legumes that thrive in disturbed sites in arid and marginal habitats. It is mostly a prostrate plant with long divided leaves with numerous pea-like, purple to white flowers. These mature into beaked legume pods that have a groove along the side. The pods are often red and spotted. (B) *Oxytropis sericea* or white point locoweed. This locoweed is also a perennial native that grows clusters of legume-like leaves with several flowering stalks that can grow up to 30 cm tall. This crown is supported by a deep tap root that allows remarkable drought tolerance. It has white flowers that produce a legume pod containing hundreds of dark, hard, haired, kidney-shaped seeds that can survive decades in the soil. White point locoweed's dormant soil seed bank and its deep tap root allow it to persist in difficult habitats where others fail. (C) *Astragalus mollissimus* or wooly locoweed. This is also a perennial that grows up to nearly 1 m tall with hair-covered leaves and stems. The leaves are pinnate with oval hairy leaflets. The flowers are pink to purple, and they mature into egg-shaped pods 2 to 3 cm in diameter. Wooly locoweed lacks the drought tolerance of white point locoweed, so populations tend to have precipitation-associated fluctuations.

storage and neurologic disease have been demonstrated in other toxic plants including certain *Swainsona, Ipomoea, Turbina,* and *Sida* species.[5]

Locoweed poisoning causes extensive neurologic and visceral vacuolation with disruption of nearly all endocrine and reproductive functions. With extended exposure, severe cellular mannosidosis develops with clinical signs becoming apparent after 10 to 14 days of exposure. Early signs in horses include reluctance to move and loss of condition and emaciation. The first neurologic signs include weakness, mild proprioceptive deficits, and minimal intention tremors that are only noticeable when animals are forced to move and navigate obstacles. With continued poisoning, horses develop severe neurologic signs including depression, disorientation and obvious loss of proprioception, excitability, irregular gait often including hypermetria, and incoordination. Horses eventually become anorexic and recumbent as they are often reluctant or have difficulty in rising. Poisoning is generally not fatal until the neurologically compromised animals encounter some mishap.[6]

Most locoweed-poisoned horses do not have specific gross lesions. Common secondary changes include polycystic ovarian disease, abortion, cachexia, and marked atrophy of adipose tissue (**Fig. 2A–E**). Microscopic lesions are remarkable and characteristic of poisoning. These are described as widespread visceral and neurologic cytoplasmic vacuolation. Horses are unique as they develop severe neurologic vacuolation that is most severe in cerebellar Purkinje cells. The most consistent cerebellar lesions are seen in the central cerebellar lobe (see **Fig. 2A–E**). Horses also develop extensive vacuolation of visceral and endocrine tissues including hepatocyte vacuolation, and thyroid follicular epithelial vacuolation.[7] The visceral lesions are reversible, and they quickly recover within weeks of discontinued exposure.[8] Resolution of neuronal vacuolation is slower, and if severe, often results in neuronal necrosis and permanent neuronal loss. Repeated poisonings are cumulative as poisoned horses lose condition until they are culled. Previously poisoned animals become reproductively functional within several months; however, as most of the neurologic lesions are permanent, poisoned animals should not be used for work.[8,9]

Diagnosis depends on identifying exposure and ingestion with supporting clinical signs and microscopic lesions. As some locoweed populations have varying endophyte infections and subsequent swainsonine concentrations, plant sampling and analysis may be indicated. As endophyte infections are transmitted vertically in the seed, once populations are identified as toxic, the endophyte infection rates change little. Chemical detection of serum and tissue swainsonine concentrations can identify animals currently ingesting locoweeds. However, swainsonine clearance is rapid with a half-life of about 20 hours. Consequently, samples collected from animals removed from locoweed-infested ranges several days prior to testing will not contain detectable serum swainsonine concentrations.

NITROTOXINS

Over 250 nitrotoxin-containing *Astragalus* species have been identified in North America. Other nitrotoxin-containing plants include species of the *Cornoilla, Indigofera, Lotus,* and *Hippocrepis* genera and several fungi from *Arthrinium, Aspergillus,* and *Penicillium* genera.[10] Nitrotoxins are generally found in plants as glycosides. A common glycoside is miserotoxin, the β-D-glucoside of 3-nitro-1-propanol. Glycosides are not directly toxic, but become toxic via hydrolysis into nitropropanol and nitropropionic acid (NPA). NPA has been shown to irreversibly inhibit succinate dehydrogenase and subsequently block oxidative phosphorylation.[11] As nitrotoxins also oxidize

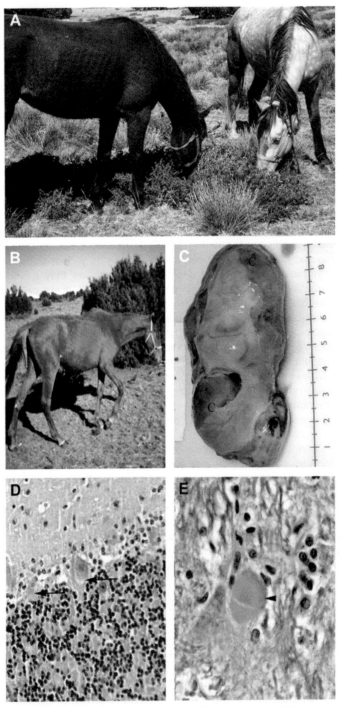

Fig. 2. (*A*) Horses readily eat locoweeds consequently exposure should be avoided. Continuous exposure for several weeks is required to develop disease. (*B*) Anorexia, weight loss, and loss of condition are early signs of poisoning. This horse was exposed to locoweed for

hemoglobin, methemoglobinemia has been used as an indicator of poisoning. Methemoglobin does not appear to contribute to the neurologic disease as prevention of its formation does not alter disease progression. Gamma-aminobutyric acid (GABA)ergic neurons common in the basal ganglia appear to be especially sensitive to NPA damage. It is suggested that NPA toxicity accentuates glutamate toxicity, possibly through the N-methyl-D-aspartate receptor.[12] Livestock poisoned by NPA often develop rear limb incoordination, proprioceptive deficits, weakness, and altered gait resulting in interference or clacker heels. Histologically, they have necrosis of the thalamus, patchy cerebellar Purkinje cell necrosis, spongiosis of the white tracts in the globus pallidus, distension of the lateral ventricles, and Wallerian degeneration of the ventral and lateral columns of the spinal cord and sciatic nerves. NPA toxicity in horses is poorly described. One potential NPA intoxication in horses may be Australian "Birdsville disease" caused by ingestion of *Indigofera linnaei*. Affected horses are weak, depressed, uncoordinated, and may shiver, twitch, and sway when standing. Histologic changes have not been completely characterized but there also appears to be neuronal degeneration and necrosis in the basal ganglia.[13] Diagnosis is largely made by correlating exposure to plants with clinical and histologic changes. Chronic poisoning is difficult to identify microscopically as the lesion primarily affects neurons in the basal ganglia that secondarily alters cerebellar Purkinje cell populations.

Conium maculatum and *Cicuta* spp. (poison and water hemlock) both have the potential to poison horses, but the mechanisms of poisoning and the conditions that lead to poisoning are very different (**Fig. 3**A–E).

Both hemlocks are unpalatable and though poisoning has been reported for both, poison hemlock poisoning is more frequent in horses. This generally occurs in the early spring when other forages are coarse, dried stems, or completely depleted and poison hemlock is the only green plant available (see **Fig. 3**B). The toxins, conine and gamma-coniceine, are nicotinic agonists causing muscle tremors, hypersalivation, incoordination, dyspnea, increased defecation and urination, and death.[14] As a result of the way horses eat, they often develop malaise and mild symptoms before they consume a fatal dose. Such sublethal poisoning is usually characterized by weakness resulting in recumbency and obvious mental depression. Often such horses will have a musty or mouse-like smell to their breath. Horses that survive the initial nicotinic effects can recover over 6 to 10 hours if they are allowed to calmly rest. If they become anxious, tranquilizers may be indicated.

As poison hemlock often invades into fields, leaves and stems may contaminate hay and silage. The seeds are also highly toxic and can contaminate cereal grains. However, coniine is relatively unstable and it degrades over several months in most hay and prepared feeds. Fresh plant material is uniformly toxic, and poisonings commonly occur when other livestock are fed contaminated fresh, chopped forages.

Water hemlock (*Cicuta maculata*- see **Fig. 3**C) is a highly toxic, convulsive plant. Poisoning in horses is uncommon, and there are few reports compared with poisoning

---

8 weeks and developed neurologic disease. Notice the rough hair coat and loss of condition. (C) This is the ovary from a horse that was dosed with ground *Astragalus lentiginosus* to obtain swainsonine doses of 0.5 mg swainsonine/Kg body weight/day for 6 weeks. Notice the large follicular cysts (C). The mare had severe neurologic disease and constantly demonstrated behavioral estrus. (D) Cerebellum of a horse that was dosed with ground *Astragalus lentiginosus* to obtain doses of 1.5 mg swainsonine/Kg body weight/day for 6 weeks. Notice the swollen Purkinje cells (*arrow*) that contain granular cytoplasmic vesicles. (E) Cerebellar crus of the same horse that had a large eosinophilic spheroid (axonal dystrophy *arrowhead*).

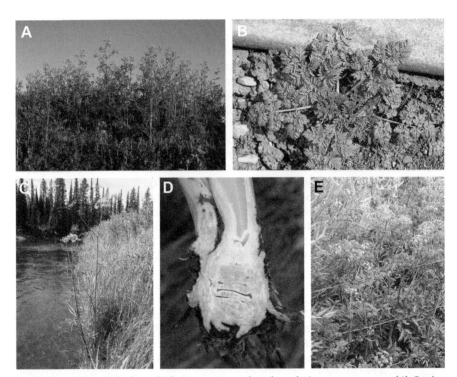

Fig. 3. These 2 hemlocks have little in common other than their common name. (*A*) *Conium maculatum* (Poison hemlock*)* is a biennial or annual carrot-like plant from Europe and North Africa. In Australia, Western Asia, and North and South America, it is a hardy invasive weed that invades and often dominates pastures, fields, and rangelands. It has carrot-like leaves that extend along the stem that grows up to 2.5 m tall. The stem is hollow, glaborous, and often has red to purple spots and patches. The flowers are small clusters, and each has 5 petals. (*B*) The first-year poison hemlock sprouts in early spring before other plants. This stage is most commonly eaten by horses when other forages are not available. (*C*) *Cicuta maculata* and others (Water hemlock) are perennials that tend to grow in moist environments along streams and ditches. The stem is hollow with root tubers that are multichambered and filled with yellowish oily liquid (*D*). The alternative leaves are lanceolate and serrate. The flowers are small green to white umbel shaped that develop into numerous cylindrical greenish fruits (*E*).

in other livestock.[15] Poisoning generally occurs in late summer when other forages are depleted, and the only green forages are in moist soils adjacent to rivers, streams, or irrigation ditches. Water hemlock toxin, cicutoxin, is in all plant parts, but is most concentrated in the tuberous root (see **Fig. 3**D) and the mature seeds (see **Fig. 3**E). Cicutoxin is a non-competitive (GABA) receptor antagonist resulting in neurologic hyperactivity convulsive seizures. Signs begin within minutes of ingestion, and they include nausea, vomiting, colic, tremors, confusion, weakness, and seizures followed by respiratory failure and ventricular fibrillation. Diazepam is often recommended to reduce seizures. Activated charcoal may reduce further toxin absorption. Diagnosis is made by chemical isolation of the toxin in gastric contents, blood, or urine. Recovery may take several days, and some neurologic changes may persist for months post exposure.

Quercus spp. (Oaks) include hundreds of species of shrubs and trees. All are considered toxic with seedlings, early bud growth, and acorns being the cause of most intoxications. Poisoning generally occurs in early spring or fall when toxic acorns or early growth are available and alternative forages are limited. Toxicity has been attributed to tannins; however, purified tannins are not very toxic suggesting there is probably an unidentified toxic component. Tannins are polyphenolic compounds that cross-link proteins and other macromolecules resulting in gastrointestinal epithelial and renal tubular epithelial degeneration and necrosis. Initial signs of poisoning include lethargy, constipation, tenesmus, polydipsia, polyuria, and a brown discoloration of the urine. These are followed by hemorrhagic diarrhea, abdominal pain, rumen atony, and anorexia. Oak-induced renal disease is characterized by isosthenuria, glucosuria, proteinuria, and hematuria with serum biochemical changes of hyperkalemia, hyperphosphatemia, azotemia, and hypercreatinemia. Postmortem changes include hemorrhagic debris mixed with leaf and acorn shell material in the stomach and proximal intestine; hemorrhagic enterocolitis with blood-filled intestines; and swollen and reddened kidneys. Microscopic lesions are characterized by diffuse cortical renal tubular degeneration and necrosis with tubular casts.[16]

Diagnosis is made by associating the clinical presentation, pathologic findings, and evidence of ingestion. Chemical detection of tannin metabolites has limited use as they are readily eliminated and often undetectable in tissues. Poisoning can be prevented by limiting exposure to oak materials by cleaning up branches and acorns in or near paddocks. Treatment is symptomatic and supportive for hemorrhagic diarrhea and renal damage.

Oxalate-Containing Plants can contain soluble or insoluble oxalates. Insoluble oxalates are generally present as calcium oxalate crystals in plants. These crystals are very irritating to mucosal membranes, and when eaten they damage the oral cavity and gastrointestinal tract. Such plants are not palatable and generally avoided; however, if horses are forced to eat them, they develop oral mucosal hyperemia, swelling, and marked hypersalivation. Soluble oxalates include sodium and potassium oxalate and oxalic acid. These are quickly absorbed and cause systemic poisoning. Only a few species of the *Agave*, *Beta*, *Bassia*, *Chenopodium*, *Halogeton*, *Oxalis*, *Rhuem*, *Rumex*, *Sarcobatus*, and *Setaria* genera contain enough soluble oxalates to be reported as toxic. Acute poisoning (usually seen in plants with >10% soluble oxalates) usually results in fatal nephrosis and renal failure. Such massive poisoning is relatively rare in horses and other monogastric animals. These are more likely to develop chronic poisoning (low oxalate doses for extended durations). As calcium supplementation does not alter acute poisoning and nephrosis, additional mechanisms of toxicity were found to contribute to nephrosis. An oxalate metabolite, calcium oxalate monohydrate (COM), damages mitochondrial function, impairing oxidative phosphorylation.[17] COM crystals also alter membrane structure and function resulting in physical damage and increased reactive oxygen species that further damage cells.[18]

Plants associated with oxalate poisoning in horses include buffel, pangola, setaria, kikuyu (**Fig. 4**A–C), green panic, guinea, signal, and purple pigeon grasses.[19] Chronic poisoning, as most often seen in horses, most often results in secondary hyperparathyroidism resulting in bony resorption with secondary osseous proliferation and dysplasia. Oxalates effectively bind and sequester calcium and magnesium resulting in functional deficiencies including altered neurologic function.[20] Poisoned horses show weakness, stiffness, intermittent lameness, inability to work, weight loss, and swelling of the osseous proliferation of flat bones especially of the head. Grossly and histologically they develop fibrous osteodystrophy with swelling of the nasal bones, maxilla, and mandible (see **Fig. 4**B and C). Associated histologic changes include increased osteoclast activity, dystrophic mineralization with proliferation of fibrous connective tissue.[21] Treatments are symptomatic including calcium and electrolyte

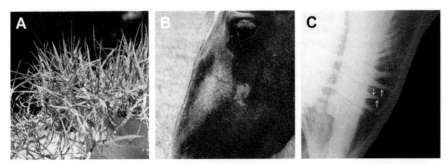

Fig. 4. (A) Oxylate-containing kikeuegrass (*Penisetum clendestrum*) in Hawaii that was associated with fibrous osteodystrophy in horses. (B) Horse with oxalate-associated fibrous osteodystrophy causing swelling of the maxilla and mandible. (C) Radiograph of the maxilla, mandible, and teeth of a horse with oxalate-associated fibrous osteodystrophy. Note the radiodense proliferations that expand from the dental roots.

replacement. Limiting exposure and reducing risk of poisoning by identifying oxalate-containing plants and by analyzing oxalate concentrations of potentially toxic plant populations is recommended.[19,22]

Solanum spp. (*Nightshades*) (*S. rostratum* [buffalo bur], *S. ptycanthum* [black nightshade], *S. dulcamara* [bittersweet], *S. elaeagnifolium* [silverleaf nightshade], *S. carolinense* [Carolina horse nettle], *S. dimidiatum* [western horse nettle], and *S. triflorum* (cutleaf nightshade)) are a diverse group of toxic plants resulting in several poisoning syndromes. Several contain steroidal glycoalkaloids that cause severe gastroenteritis. Others contain cholinesterase inhibitors that cause neurologic disease. The most common toxin is the alkaloid solanine, a potent mucosal irritant resulting in severe stomatitis and gastroenteritis. Solanine concentrations are highest in the berries that often poison both livestock and humans. Signs include anorexia, increased salivation and slobbering, abdominal pain, diarrhea, dilation of pupils, dullness, depression, weakness, progressive paralysis, prostration, and rarely death. Treatment generally is symptomatic and most animals quickly recover when exposure is discontinued.[14]

Convolvulus arvensis (field bindweed or morning glory) is an invasive, noxious weed that invades and often dominates pastures, paddocks, and disturbed areas (**Fig. 5**). Poisoning appears to be exclusive to horses. Disease occurs when horses graze bindweed for weeks or months. Affected horses have diarrhea, colic, gastrointestinal ulceration and intestinal thickening, and fibrosis. Attempts to isolate the cause have been frustrating. Convolvulin, a resinoid, and several tropane alkaloids have been suggested, but have not been confirmed experimentally.[23] More work is needed to better understand this poisoning, determine the pathogenesis, and identify methods to avoid poisoning.

TRIFOLIUM HYBRIDUM (ALSIKE CLOVER)

Alsike clover, a perennial legume, is a short-lived forage plant included in many pasture-seed mixes. It often escapes cultivation dominating margins, fence rows, and ditches. This clover has 15 to 70 cm tall erect, ascending stems and flat, oval leaves (~0.4 cm × 0.3 cm) in leaflets of 3. It has many flowers (0.25 cm) with white to pink petals that fade to reddish-brown. It is most common in low, moist meadows and pastures. It was originally used as legume forage for hay, pasture, and soil improvement. Several toxins have been suspected, but none have been proven. Toxicity may be

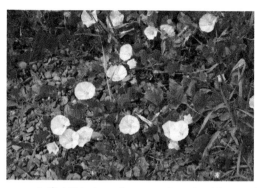

Fig. 5. *Convulvulus arvensis* (field bindweed, or morning glory) is a noxious invasive perennial weed. It is prostrate, with alternative leaves and white, funnel-shaped flowers. It has both seeds and extensive rhizome systems, making it difficult to control.

related to environmental conditions as those conducive to mold or aflatoxin production increase incidence. Three syndromes have been identified in horses. No other species is known to be susceptible. The first, "dew poisoning," is characterized by photosensitivity (sunburn), colic and diarrhea, depression, or excitation. The second, "big liver disease" is severe or recurrent liver disease seen clinically as icterus, weight loss, central nervous system (CNS) depression, anorexia, incoordination, dark and discolored urine, and an enlarged fibrotic liver. Chronic exposure (weeks to months) is generally required before horses develop liver disease. The third syndrome is associated with excessive salivation or slobbering, when horses eat clover that is infected with a fungus that causes brown leaf spot. Horses stop slobbering when exposure is discontinued.[24] Treatment includes removing horses from exposure to the plant, treating photosensitivity, and supportive care. Recovered animals often are hepatic cripples and more susceptible to liver failure or other liver diseases. It is recommended that alsike clover not be included in pasture seed mixes for horses.

Centauria solstitialis, C. repens, and *C. melitensis* (yellow-star thistle, knapweed, and Malta star thistle **Fig. 6**A and B). Knapweed/yellow-star thistle poisoning are considered diseases of neglect, occurring in horses, donkeys, and mules that have limited feed and are forced to eat the plants for several months. Some horses develop a taste for knapweed, and they may continue eating it even when supplemented with other forage. At cumulative doses of 50% to 200% of their body weight over 30 to 90 days, horses develop dysfunction of facial, mouth, and throat nerves and muscles.[14] This poisoning has been called "chewing disease" (horses chew but can't swallow). Knapweed-induced facial muscle hypertonicity is seen clinically as "smiling," tongue lolling, protruding tongue, and head tossing. Poisoning impairs the ability to drink as thirsty horses, trying to drink will submerge their muzzle and face in the water and splash with no apparent satisfaction. Early neurologic signs progress to lethargy, loss of interest in food, dehydration, malnutrition, difficulty breathing, incoordination, muscle tremors, and severe depression. Knapweed and yellow star thistle induce specific microscopic lesions in the substancia nigra and globus pallidus. The neurons in these nuclei include many motor neurons of the vagus, hypoglossal, and facial cranial nerves that innervate the tongue, mouth, and face. This unique lesion, called nigropallidal encephalomalacia, is unique to this disease. The long exposures and lack of a smaller animal model make it difficult to positively identify the toxin. As there is no treatment and the disease is irreversible, it is best to avoid exposure to the plants

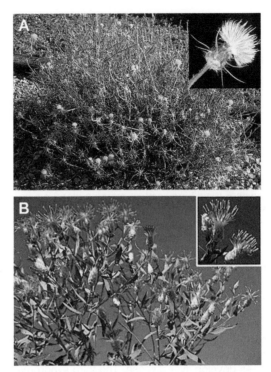

Fig. 6. (*A*) *Centauria solstitialis* (yellow-star thistle) is a Mediterranean weed that has become established in many western and southern states. It is invasive and dominates many roadsides and disturbed areas. Yellow-star thistle is a branching annual with finely haired leaves that are lobed basally and linear on the stem. The disc flowers are yellow, and the bracts are tipped with stiff yellow spines. (*B*) *Centaurea repens* (Russian knapweed) invades fields, pastures, and roadsides. It is a persistent, noxious weed that grows in all soil types, spreads by both seeds and rhizomes, and is allelopathic. A perennial, Russian knapweed is generally erect (~1 m tall) and the stems are covered with fine hairs. The leaves are alternate with serrated margins. The flowers form thistle-like heads (1 cm) and vary from white to purple. The paper-like bracts have no spines. Most seeds remain on the seed head, which is easily spread by animals. (Both photos are courtesy of Anthony Knight.)

for prolonged periods. Any animals that willingly eat these plants should be removed from knapweed-containing or yellow star thistle-containing pastures or ranges.

  Vicia villosa (hairy vetch), *V. lavenworthii* (lavenworth vetch) are introduced European plants that grow across North America. These vetches have become established as weeds that grow in waste areas and along roadsides. Hairy vetch is a prostrate or climbing annual that can get up to 2 m long or tall. Leaves have 10 to 20, 2.5 cm-long leaflets with tendrils at the leaf ends. Flowers are purple to red with 20 to 60 flowers on 1 side of the flowering spike. The flowers form 2 to 3 cm seed pods that contain small, hard seeds. Vetch is problematic in late spring and midsummer. The toxin has not been identified and the development of disease is poorly understood. Poisoning generally affects black horses by introducing a multi-systemic granulomatous disease. The granulomatous reaction suggests this is most likely an allergic or hypersensitivity disease. Disease is sporadic, and clinical signs include fever, dermal edema, and other signs depending on the tissue or organs affected (skin, lymph node, lungs, kidneys, liver, heart, gastrointestinal tract, skeletal muscle, and eyes).[14]

Poisoning usually is fatal. Because there is no proven treatment and the disease is irreversible, avoiding exposure is essential.

Photosensitization: Photosensitization is common in horses, and can be attributed to various diseases and toxins. It is light-induced dermatitis caused by photodynamic agents or chromophores in the skin, resulting in heightened sensitivity of the skin to sunlight. Chromophores absorb light energy and transfer it to adjacent proteins, nucleic acids, and membranes. This energy directly damages tissues; it also generates reactive molecules and oxidative chemical reactions in dermal components. The result is epithelial cell damage, degeneration, and necrosis. As most chromophores are not cytotoxic until they are photoactivated, clinical dermatitis only develops after exposure to sunlight. Both hair and dermal pigments absorb light energy, consequently radiation-induced dermatitis is most severe in lightly pigmented areas with little hair protection — muzzle, ears, eyelids, face, tail, vulva, udder, and coronary bands. Even black, hairy animals may become affected in severe poisoning. Clinical signs include photophobia and discomfort seen as scratching and rubbing the ears, eyelids, and muzzle. Horses with white skin and relatively thin hair may develop dermatitis that impairs using tack, precluding their use. Lesions will recover with appropriate therapy and housing animals in the shade.

Plant-associated photosensitization can be primary or secondary. Primary photosensitization is caused directly by plant-associated chromophores. Secondary or hepatogenic photosensitization occurs when impaired liver function results in accumulation of phylloerythrin, a chlorophyll metabolite, that when combined with irradiation causes photosensitization.

Primary Photosensitization

Hypericum perforatum (St. John's wort, goat weed, Tipton weed, amber or Klamath weed- **Fig. 7**A) is a perennial that grows along roadsides and in meadows, pastures, rangelands, and waste places in the North American Pacific coast states and in Europe, Australia, New Zealand, and South America. It usually is found on dry, gravelly, or sandy soils in full sunshine. It may grow in dense patches or mixed among other plants where it may contaminate feeds. It is considered a noxious weed in many states. St. John's wort is dangerous at all stages of growth. Young tender shoots may attract animals in the spring. Normally, livestock will not eat mature St. John's wort if other forage is available. Signs usually appear 2 to 21 days after ingestion. The principal photodynamic toxin has been identified as hypericin, an endophyte-produced compound used historically as an herbal remedy.[25]

Fagopyrum esculentum and F. tataricum (North American buckwheat) are perennial subshrubs or vines with simple, alternate leaves and cream and white flowers. They grow up to 0.6 m tall in disturbed soils along field margins and fences. Native to Asia, they were initially imported as cover crops that have been replaced by less toxic plants making poisoning mostly historical. Buckwheats contain hypericin-like toxins (fagopyrin, photofagopyrin, and pseudohypericin).[14]

Furanocoumarin-containing plants: *Cymopterus watsonii* (Spring parsley- **Fig. 7**B) poisons horses in early spring when it is often the only green forage available. In early summer, it matures and senesces. It grows in pastures and rangelands on well-drained soils at elevations of 1500 to 3500 m[26]

Ammi majus (Bishop's Weed) is a carrot-like weed found in central and southern states. It grows 20 to 80 cm tall with 3-pinnately compound or dissected leaves with terminal linear to lanceolate leaflets. Flowers are compound with small white petals. Originally from Eurasia, they are found on waste areas and along roadways and fence lines. Most poisonings are reported in lambs and calves.[27]

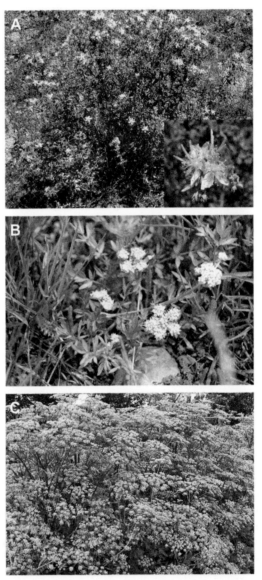

Fig. 7. (*A*) *Hypericum perforatum* (St. John's wort) is a smooth-branched, erect plant that may reach a height of 2 m. The leaves are covered with clear, small dots that contain the toxic substance (hypericin). The flowers have 5 petals that grow in clusters; they are orange-yellow with small black dots along the edges (insert). It has expanded and now it can be found in many western states. (*B*) *Cymopterus watsonii* (Spring parsley) is a short perennial that grows 8 to 12 cm tall. It has a deep taproot that allows it considerable drought tolerance. It has parsley-like, finely divided leaves. The flowers are small white or cream colored. (*C*) *Pastinaca sativa* (Wild parsnip) has been a noxious weed in many states. It is a biennial plant that is first a rosette with hairy leaves. It grows a cream-colored edible taproot that is conical to bulbus shaped. The leaves are often twice pinnate with broad ovate leaflets with toothed margins. The flower umbellets are composed of 5 yellow petals and 5 stamens. These mature into schizocarp fruits that are brown, oval, flat, and between 4 and 8 mm long.

Thamnosma texana and *T. montana* (Dutchman's Breeches) are perennial weeds of the southwest United States. They grow up to 60 cm tall and have simple alternate leaves. Flowers are blue to yellow. They are native to dry rocky slopes.[28]

Pastinaca sativa (wild parsnip- **Fig. 7**C) poisons horses most often when it infests pastures. It can also contaminate hay. Parsnip is a Eurasian plant that can grow up to 2 m tall. The leaves are alternate, compound, and branched with jagged teeth. It flowers in early summer with hundreds of yellow flowers forming an umbel. It has a deep tap root making it somewhat drought tolerant. It often forms large patches in pastures and ranges. It contains several furanocoumarins—xanthotoxin, bergapten, isopimpinellin, imperatorin, and a putative methoxy imperatorin. Though some incidents have been attributed to wild parsnip ingestion, most lesions are associated with contact dermatitis. Cutaneous application of wild parsnip extracts produce severe photodermatitis similar to that observed in clinical poisoning.[29]

Rotting celery, parsnips, and other vegetables can be infected with fungi that produce phytoalexins (commonly xanthotoxin and tripsoralen). These cause topical or contact photosensitization/dermatitis. Phytoalexin-induced photodermatitis is most common in pigs.[30]

Secondary Photosensitization

The most common type of photosensitization in livestock is secondary. Phylloerythrin is a chlorophyll metabolite that is primarily formed by enteric microorganisms. Photosensitization caused by increased circulating and dermal phylloerythrin concentrations has been identified as hepatogenous or secondary photosensitization.[31] Phylloerythrin is absorbed from the gastrointestinal tract and carried to the liver via the portal circulation. Normally, hepatocytes conjugate phylloerythrin and excrete it in bile. However, if the liver is damaged or bile excretion is impaired, phylloerythrin accumulates, including in the skin, causing photosensitivity.

Photosensitization generally develops in horses when serum phylloerythrin concentrations are >8.0 μg/dl and serum bile acid concentrations are > 10.0 μmol/l.[31] Clinical photosensitivity requires 3 independent variables. First, liver damage and impaired biliary excretion results in phylloerythrin accumulation. Second, ingestion of adequate green forage results in intestinal chlorophyll metabolism producing abundant phylloerythrin. Some feeds and microbiomes can produce excessive phylloerythrin that overwhelms normal excretion pathways in juveniles. This appears to be the case with many idiopathic photosensitized young horses.[32] Finally, the animal must be exposed to enough sunlight to photoactivate the dermal phylloerythrin and damage dermal tissues. Temporary increase in one such variable can result in periodic or seasonal photosensitivity that eventually resolves.

Often, cholestasis is caused by intrahepatic necrosis and fibrosis. This can be caused by infectious, nutritional, or toxic etiologies. Most plants associated with secondary photosensitization have been previously reviewed (**Box 1**).

Animals with secondary or hepatogenous photosensitivity will have additional lesions of hepatic disease including jaundice, hepatic encephalopathy, hyperbilirubinemia, and increased serum bile acids and enzyme activities (sorbitol dehydrogenase, glutamate dehydrogenase, aspartate dehydrogenase, alkaline phosphatase). Percutaneous liver biopsies can be very helpful to evaluate the cause of liver damage.

Managing photosensitivity is done by removing the photodynamic agent, decreasing exposure to sunlight, and treating the dermal and possible hepatic lesions. This may require changing feed, pasture, and housing. Irradiation-induced dermatitis is generally best treated by protecting horses from the sun with masks or stalling them in the shade. Topical antimicrobial ointments and lotions are helpful in managing the

---

Box 1
Plants associated with secondary photosensitization in horses

Hepatotoxic plants: Dehydropyrrolizidine alkaloid (PA) containing plants, cockleburs, *Lantana* species, certain clovers

Cholestastic plants: Crystalline choleangitis- *Panicum antidotale* (blue *Panicum*), *P. coloratum* (Kleingrass), *P. dichotomiflorum* (smooth switchgrass), *P. maximum* (guineagrass), *P. miliaceum* (millet), and *P. virgatum* (switchgrass). *Tribulus* spp. (goathead or puncture vine). *Brachiaria* spp. and *Pithomyces cartarum*. *Agave lecheguilla* and *Nolina texana* (beargrass or sacahuiste), and *Narthecium ossifragum*.

---

topical lesions. If severe, animals may need fluid therapy and systemic antibiotics. Sunscreens, dermal tattooing, and protective blankets and hoods are helpful if horses cannot be removed from sunlight. Liver failure is more difficult to treat and depends largely on the cause. Inflammatory diseases such as cholangiohepatitis respond well to therapy. Toxicologic causes are more dependent on the extent of liver damage and failure. Severely damaged animals generally do not respond to treatment and may have to be euthanized.

SUMMARY

Many toxic range and pasture plants are relatively unpalatable and if adequate alternative forages are available, horses will avoid eating them. However, there are exceptions. For example, horses readily eat locoweeds regardless of forage availability. Poisoning often causes irreversible lesions that will affect animal performance throughout its life. As treatments are often difficult and poorly effective, identification of risk and avoiding exposure is the best method to avoid poisoning.

CLINICS CARE POINTS

- With the few exceptions, horses generally avoid eating free-standing poisonous plants if other forages are available.
- When alternative forages are limited, horses can eat and even develop an acceptance of toxic plants that may result in poisoning.
- As plant-induced disease can be similar to other genetic, infectious, and nutritional disease, documenting exposure and ingestion of toxic plants is an essential step in identifying poisoning. This requires complete, detailed field or range studies.
- Postmortem and microscopic studies can identify many toxic plant–induced diseases and exclude the possibility of many other diseases.
- Chemical analysis is helpful to identify toxic plant populations and analysis of ingesta or biologic samples may identify plant toxins.
- Correlation of chemical analyses or biomarkers must be correlated with clinical disease, postmortem and microscopic lesions to develop a most likely cause. and diagnosis.
- Treatment is plant-specific and generally symptomatic as antidotes are often not available.

DISCLOSURE

The authors have nothing to disclose.

REFERENCES

1. Marsh CD. Stock-poisoning plants of the range. United States Department of Agriculture Bureau Animal Industry Bulletin No 1245. pp. 22-44. 1929.
2. Marsh CD. The locoweed disease of the plains. United States Department of Agriculture Bureau Animal Industry Bulletin No. 112, 1909 Washington DC. USA. 1909.
3. Cook D, Gardner DR, Grum D, et al. Swainsonine and endophyte relationships in Astragalus mollissimus and Astragalus lentiginosus. J Agric Food Chem 2011;59: 1281-7.
4. Dorling PR, Huxtable CR, Vogel P. Lysosomal storage in Swainsona spp. toxicosis: an induced mannosidosis. Neuropathol Appl Neurobiol 1978;4:285-95.
5. Cook D, Gardner DR, Pfister JA. Swainsonine-containing plants and their relationship to endophytic fungi. J Agric Food Chem 2014;62:7326-34.
6. Stegelmeier BL, James LF, Gardner DR, et al. Locoweed (Oxytropis sericea)-induced lesions in mule deer (Odocoileius hemionus). Veterinary Pathology 2005; 42:566-78.
7. Stegelmeier BL, Lee ST, James LF, et al. The comparative pathology of locoweed poisoning in livestock, wildlife and rodents. In: Panter KE, Wierenga TL, Pfister JA, editors. Poisonous plants global research and solutions. Cambridge MA: CABI Publishing; 2007. p. 359-65.
8. Stegelmeier BL, James LF, Panter KE, et al. The pathogenesis and toxicokinetics of locoweed (Astragalus and Oxytropis spp.) poisoning in livestock. J Nat Toxins 1999;8:35-45.
9. Stegelmeier BL, Davis TZ, Welch KD, et al. The comparative pathology of locoweed poisoning in horses and other livestock. In: Riet-Correa F, Pfister JA, Schild AL, et al, editors. Poisoning by plants, myocotoxins,and related toxins. Oxfordshire UK: CABI; 2011. p. 309-10.
10. Anderson RC, Majak W, Rassmussen MA, et al. Toxicity and metabolism of the conjugates of 3-nitropropanol and 3-nitropropionic acid in forages poisonous to livestock. J Agric Food Chem 2005;53:2344-50.
11. Gould DH, Gustine DL. Basal ganglia degeneration, myelin alterations, and enzyme inhibition induced in mice by the plant toxin, 3-nitropropanoic acid. Neuropathol Appl Neurobiol 1982;8:377-93.
12. Albin RL. Basal ganglia neurotoxins. Neurol Clin 2000;18:665-80.
13. Carroll AG, Swain BJ. Birdsville disease in the central highlands area of Queensland. Aust Vet J 1983;60:316-7.
14. Burrows GE, Tyrl RJ. Toxic PLANTS of North America. Ames Iowa: Wiley Blackwell; 2013.
15. Takeda Y, Osanai R, Takahashi K, et al. Diagnosis of water hemlock poisoning in minature horses. J Jpn Vet Med Assoc 2007;60:47-51.
16. Smith S, Naylor RJ, Knowles EJ, et al. Suspecterd acorn toxicity in nine horses. Equine Vet J 2014;47:503-632.
17. McMartin KE, Wallace KB. Calcium oxalate monohydrate, a metabolite of ethylene glycol, is toxic for rat renal mitochondrial function. Toxicol Sci 2005;84: 195-200.
18. McMartin K. Are calcium oxalate crystals involved in the mechanism of acute renal failure in ethylene glycol poisoning? Clinical Toxicology (Phila) 2009;47:859-69.
19. Stewart J, Liyou O, Wilson G. Bighead in horses - not an ancient disease. Australian Equine Veterinarian 2010;29:55-62.
20. Naude TW, Naidoo V. Oxalate containing plants. In: Gupta RC, editor. Veterinary toxicology: basic and clinical principles. Boston MA: Elsevier; 2007. p. 880-91.

21. Walthall JC, McKenzie RA. Osteodystrophia fibrosa in horses at pasture in Queensland: field and laboratory observations. Aust Vet J 1976;52:11–6.
22. McKenzie RA, Gartner RJW, Blaney BJ, et al. Control of nutritional secondary hyperparathyroidism in grazing horse with calcium and phosphorous supplementation. Aust Vet J 1981;57:554–7.
23. Todd FG, Stermitz FR, Schultheis P, et al. Tropane alkaloids and toxicity of Convolvulus arvensis. Phytochemistry 1995;39:301–3.
24. Colon JL, Jackson CA, Piero Fd. Hepatic dysfunction and photodermatitis secondary to alsike clover poisoning. Compend Continuing Educ Pract Vet 1996; 18:1022–6.
25. Kusari S, Lamshoft M, Zuhlke S, et al. An endophytic fungus from Hypericum perforatum that produces hypericin. J Nat Prod 2008;71:159–62.
26. Binns W, James LF, Brooksby W. Cymopterus watsoni: a photosensitizing plant for sheep. Vet Med 1964;59:375–9.
27. Dollahite JW, Younger RL, Hoffman GO. Photosensitization in cattle and sheep caused by feeding Ammi majus (greater Ammi; Bishop's-Weed). Am J Vet Res 1978;39:193–7.
28. Oertli EH, Beier RC, Ivie GW, et al. Linear furocoumarins and other constituents from Thamnosma texana. Phytochemistry 1984;23:439–41.
29. Stegelmeier BL, Colegate SM, Knoppel EL, et al. Wild parsnip (Pastinaca sativa)-induced photosensitization. Toxicon 2019;167:60–6.
30. Beier RC. Natural pesticides and bioactive components in foods. Rev Environ Contam Toxicol 1990;113:47–137.
31. Collett MG. Bile duct lesions associated with turnip (Brassica rapa) photosensitization compared with those due to sporidesmin toxicosis in dairy cows. Veterinary Pathology 2014;51:986–91.
32. Stegelmeier BL. Equine Photosensitization. Clin Tech Equine Pract 2002;1:81–8.

Plants Causing Toxic Myopathies

Beatrice Sponseller, DVM[a],*, Tim Evans, DVM, MS, PhD[b]

KEYWORDS

- Toxic myopathy • Cardiomyopathy • Boxelder and sycamore maple • Hypoglycin A
- White snakeroot • Rayless goldenrod • Tremetol/tremetone • Benzofuran ketones

KEY POINTS

- Plant-induced toxic myopathies are highly fatal but relatively rare in the United States.
- Cases are generally more common in the fall, especially when pastures are sparse and horses may be in a negative energy balance.
- Toxin-induced cellular energy depletion appears to be the major factor in the development of toxic myopathies, resulting in necrosis of skeletal and cardiac muscles.
- There are no chemical or physiologic antidotes for these intoxications and treatment is symptomatic.
- The toxic compounds associated with these intoxications are excreted in the milk.

INTRODUCTION TO PLANTS ASSOCIATED WITH TOXIC MYOPATHIES

Seasonal pasture myopathy (SPM) and atypical myopathy (AM) associated with box-elder maple and sycamore maple, respectively, as well as intoxications involving white snakeroot and potentially rayless goldenrod (no naturally occurring cases documented) are examples of toxic, nonexertional myopathies. These intoxications occur sporadically and are generally associated with poor prognoses. Both SPM/AM and white snakeroot intoxications, as well as possible intoxications involving *Isocoma* species, represent potential diagnostic challenges. This is especially true if veterinary health professionals are not fully aware of the toxic potential of the plants involved in these diseases and/or the nutritional considerations, weather conditions, and geographic locations, as well as other potentially predisposing factors. This review will be divided into two, separate sections discussing SPM/AM and white snakeroot/rayless goldenrod intoxication, respectively, intended to provide the information necessary to diagnose, treat, and prevent these conditions.

[a] Department of Veterinary Clinical Sciences, College of Veterinary Medicine, Iowa State University, 1809 South Riverside Drive, Ames, IA 50011, USA; [b] Department of Biomedical Sciences, College of Veterinary Medicine and MU Extension, University of Missouri, W226 Veterinary Medicine Building, 1520 East Rollins Street, Columbia, MO 65211, USA
* Corresponding author.
E-mail address: beatrice@iastate.edu

Vet Clin Equine 40 (2024) 45–59
https://doi.org/10.1016/j.cveq.2023.11.001
0749-0739/24/© 2023 Elsevier Inc. All rights reserved.

SEASONAL PASTURE MYOPATHY/ATYPICAL MYOPATHY—INTRODUCTION/ BACKGROUND
Roles of Boxelder Maple and Sycamore Maple

Boxelder maple (*Acer negundo*, ash-leaved maple, box elder) and sycamore maple (*A pseudoplatanus*) are deciduous, flowering trees that belong to the Sapindaceae (soap-berry) family. Boxelder maple is native to North America while sycamore maple is native to Europe and Western Asia.[1,2] Boxelder maple is a medium-sized tree that typically grows 15 to 23 m tall and, in contrast to other maple species, has compound leaves with generally 3 leaflets, resembling ash leaves.[3] It grows preferentially in hollows along streams. The up-to-35-m-tall sycamore maple (**Fig. 1**A) has large, 5-lobed leaves. It is shade tolerant and often dominates mixed deciduous forests in cool and humid environments. The sycamore maple is often found on steep rocky slopes, ravines, and screes.[2] Once mature, both maple species flower in the spring and female trees produce abundant fruit in the form of hanging clusters of paired, winged seeds (samaras, helicopter seeds) in late summer (**Fig. 1**B and C).[2,3] Ripe seeds fall from autumn until spring and, due to their winged nature, are widely dispersed by the wind.

Role of Hypoglycin A and its Toxic Metabolites in Seasonal Pasture Myopathy/Atypical Myopathy

Ingestion of the seeds or seedlings of the boxelder maple or the sycamore maple has been associated with the development of highly fatal, nonexertional rhabdomyolysis, predominantly in horses at pasture. Cases typically occur in the fall, and in Europe, where larger outbreaks are common, also in the subsequent spring. The clinical diseases referred to as SPM in North America and AM in Europe have been linked to the toxic, nonproteinogenic, branched-chain amino acid (BCAA), hypoglycin A (HGA, L-α-amino-methylenecyclopropylpropionic acid).[4-6] Following ingestion, HGA is metabolized in the mitochondrial matrix in a 2-step enzymatic process of transamination and oxidative carboxylation, similar to other BCAAs.[7] The resulting toxic metabolite methylenecyclopropylacetyl-CoA (MCPA-CoA) inhibits multiple flavin adenine

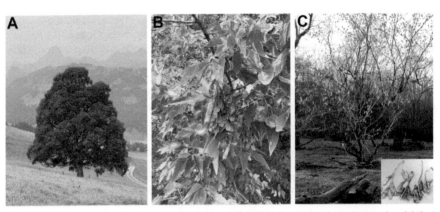

Fig. 1. A sycamore maple (*Acer pseudoplatanus*) growing in a pasture in Switzerland (*A*). A boxelder maple (*Acer negundo*) in North America is shown with its foliage still present and bearing seed-containing samaras (*B*), and (*C*) shows another boxelder maple growing in a sparse fall pasture in North America. The inset in (*C*) shows another image of seed-containing samaras. (Image courtesy Figure (A) MC de Laubarède Acer pseudoplatanus - Trees and Shrubs Online; and [B] Dr. Stephanie Valberg, Professor emeritus, Michigan State University.)

dinucleotide (FAD)–dependent mitochondrial acyl-coenzyme A dehydrogenases that catalyze the first step of fatty acid ß-oxidation and are involved in amino acid catabolism.[8] Methylenecyclopropylglycine (MCPG), a homolog of MCPA present in lower concentrations than HGA in both maple species, may contribute to the pathogenesis through in vivo formation of the toxic metabolite methylenecyclopropylformyl-CoA.[9,10] The latter is a potent inhibitor of enoyl-CoA hydratases, the catalysts of the second step of fatty acid ß-oxidation.[11]

CLINICAL ASPECTS OF SEASONAL PASTURE MYOPATHY/ATYPICAL MYOPATHY
Pathogenesis and Clinical Signs

Disruption of cellular energy metabolism by HGA and its toxic metabolites predominantly affects highly oxidative (type 1) myofibers, abundant in postural and respiratory muscles, and cardiac myocytes, which depend highly on fatty acids as an energy source. Inhibited mitochondrial ß-oxidation leads to cellular energy depletion and accumulation of fatty acids with resulting acute myonecrosis and lipid storage myopathy.[4,12] Common clinical signs include acute muscular weakness, stiffness, muscle tremors, prolonged recumbency, myoglobinuria, depression, congested mucous membranes, sweating and tachycardia. Signs of colic are common and may be severe. Cardiac arrhythmias, dyspnea, dysphagia, esophageal obstruction, bladder distention, and dysuria may also occur.[4,12–14] Mortality rates from 70% to 90% have been reported, with natural death or euthanasia most common in the first 2 to 3 days of onset of clinical signs.[12]

Diagnosis of Seasonal Pasture Myopathy/Atypical Myopathy

Antemortem diagnosis

Horses with clinical signs of SPM/AM have markedly elevated serum activities of creatine kinase (CK) and aspartate aminotransferase (AST), reflecting skeletal muscle necrosis. Cardiac troponin 1 concentrations are often elevated due to myocardial injury.[14,15] Hyperglycemia and hypocalcemia are hallmarks of SPM/AM. Metabolic profile analysis shows elevated serum acylcarnitines and urine organic acids, characteristic of the underlying multiple acyl-CoA dehydrogenase deficiency (MADD), and is available through human laboratories that screen newborns for an inherited form of MADD.[13,16,17] Documentation of a MADD-specific acylcarnitine profile supports a diagnosis of SPM/AM while a subset of measured acylcarnitines may be of prognostic value.[18] A definitive diagnosis is reached by documenting HGA or conjugates of its toxic metabolite (MCPA) in the serum, urine, or muscle of affected horses.[4,5,19] MCPA-carnitine is the most prevalent HGA metabolite in serum while MCPA-glycine is prevalent in urine and may be the primary detoxification metabolite. Analytical procedures using a variety of different liquid chromatographic separation methods, as well as mass spectrometric detection, have been optimized in recent years to offer a rapid and affordable diagnostic test for SPM/AM and are commercially available in some European countries.[20] Inclusion of MCPG and its metabolites in the diagnostic analysis may help improve the understanding of the toxicologic processes associated with boxelder and sycamore maple poisoning.[9,10]

Postmortem diagnosis

Postmortem evaluation shows widespread areas of pallor and, in some cases, hemorrhage of predominantly postural and respiratory muscles. Intercostal muscles, diaphragm, and muscles of the neck and shoulders are consistently affected, but lesions may also be present in the masseters, tongue, and muscles of the back and hindquarters.[21,22] Histopathologic evaluation reveals multifocal, monophasic acute myocyte degeneration morphologically consistent with Zenker's necrosis, predominantly affecting type 1 myofibers. Inflammatory response is minimal, with occasional slight macrophage and/or neutrophil infiltration of affected myofibers. Excessive intramyo-fiber lipid storage is a consistent finding in horses with SPM/AM and can be documented using histochemical staining for neutral triglycerides with Oil Red O. Similar gross and histopathologic changes may be present in the myocardium of horses with SPM/AM.[13,21,22]

Differential Diagnoses

Other syndromes involving severe rhabdomyolysis such as recurrent exertional rhabdomyolysis, polysaccharide storage myopathy, postanaesthetic myopathy, immune-mediated myopathy, clostridial myonecrosis, and toxic myopathy due to plant toxins from *Ageratina altissima* (*Eupatorium rugosum* or white snakeroot) or *Cassia occidentalis* (coffee weed or coffee senna) should be considered as differentials and ruled out, if necessary.[21–23] Other known causes of severe rhabdomyolysis, which should be considered as possible differential diagnoses for SPM/AM, include nutritional myodegeneration and malignant hyperthermia.[23] Conditions involving hypovolemic or endo-toxemic shock, especially colic, are also potential differential diagnoses for SPM/AM. Conditions leading to abnormal gait and, particularly, recumbency, including laminitis, various neurologic diseases, ionophore intoxication, pleuropneumonia, hyperkalemic periodic paralysis, and hypocalcemia, can also present with signs similar to those of SPM/AM.[21–23] In addition, the acute form of equine grass sickness is another condition that has several similarities with AM in regard to clinical signs, epidemiology, and associated risk factors.[23]

Hypoglycin A Concentrations in Boxelder and Sycamore Maples and Predisposing Factors for Seasonal Pasture Myopathy/Atypical Myopathy

The HGA concentration in boxelder and sycamore maple seeds is highly variable, with a reported range of 3 to 160 µg/seed for boxelder and 25 to 3683 µg/g of seed for syc-amore maple.[4,24] This variation may be due to differences in the stage of seed maturity and environmental factors such as rainfall and temperature.[25] Variable amounts of HGA have also been reported in boxelder maple seedlings and leaves.[24,26,27] Despite what appears to be a dose-dependent action of HGA (based on estimated consumption, clinical signs, and serum concentrations of HGA and its metabolites), the toxic threshold for HGA ingestion and serum MCPA concentration in horses likely varies, depending on the individual's energy balance and reliance on the ß-oxidation pathway for energy production. Cases of SPM/AM typically occur in the fall when there is an abundance of seeds and pastures are characterized by sparse vegetation.[21–23] A combination of inclement weather and reduced availability of feedstuffs may result in a negative energy balance and increased mobilization of fatty acids as an energy source, requiring use of the metabolic pathways inhibited by HGA and its toxic metabolites, thereby predisposing horses to clinical manifestation of SPM/AM.[23] Furthermore, horses with existing increased energy needs, such as young, growing animals (<3 years of age) or horses with a poor body condition score, appear to have a higher risk of developing AM.[14,18,21–23]

Treatment and Prevention

Treatment

Treatment of horses with SPM/AM is symptomatic and should include intravenous (IV) fluid therapy for hydration and correction of electrolyte and acid-base imbalances, provision of glucose to stimulate carbohydrate metabolism, and antioxidants (vitamin

C, vitamin E/selenium) to protect cells from increased free radicals produced with fatty acid oxidation disorders.[28,29] Riboflavin (vitamin B2) is a precursor of FAD, a cofactor of acyl-CoA dehydrogenases inhibited by HGA, and supplementation may enhance residual enzyme activity. Carnitine promotes fatty acid metabolism, may act as a detoxifying agent, and is a recommended treatment in human MADD.[30,31] The effect and safety of carnitine supplementation in horses with SPM/AM has not been documented. Restricting movement and decreasing stress of affected horses are imperative. Analgesics and muscle relaxants are often indicated due to an appreciable amount of pain associated with rhabdomyolysis. Oral administration of charcoal and/or a laxative within 2 days of ingestion of the plant material may reduce intestinal absorption of toxins.[30] This could also serve as a preventative measure in cograzing horses that may have ingested HGA-containing maple seeds or seedlings.[32] Documentation of HGA in blood confirms exposure of cograzing horses to the toxin.[33] Elevated serum MCPA-carnitine concentration and CK activity have also been documented in subclinical cases, albeit to a lesser degree compared to clinically affected horses.[34]

Prevention
In Europe, where large outbreaks of AM in the fall are common, cases are often observed in the subsequent spring, likely due to ingestion of maple seedlings. Standing water that had been in contact with seedlings may serve as an additional source of HGA.[35] Pasture management in the form of herbicidal spraying is ineffective in reducing HGA concentrations while mowing may temporarily increase HGA content in dying seedlings. The best preventative measure is to prohibit horses from having access to pastures with boxelder or sycamore maples and, since dried seeds and seedlings retain toxicity, to refrain from producing hay from these pastures.[36] Early detection of abnormal parameters in affected animals is not only of value in disease prevention in unaffected pasture mates but also in the management of subclinical SPM/AM in cograzing horses.[34]

Miscellaneous Information Regarding Hypoglycin A and Seasonal Pasture Myopathy/Atypical Myopathy

Mammary excretion of hypoglycin A and its toxic metabolites
Vertical transmission of HGA and its toxic metabolites has been described in a 6-hour-old as well as an 8-day-old foal, with one mare suffering and recovering from AM in the 6th month of gestation and the other mare showing clinical signs of AM at the time of presentation with her foal.[37,38] Detection of HGA and its metabolites in the mare's milk suggests transmammary transfer of toxins, although a transplacental component cannot be ruled out.[38,39] Sporadic samples of frozen commercial mare's milk labeled for human consumption and raw cow's milk have also tested positive for HGA and its metabolites and may pose a food safety concern.[38,40]

Species susceptibility
SPM/AM associated with HGA and its toxic metabolites predominantly affects horses and occasionally other equids, including donkeys and zebras.[12] Rare reports of other affected species include zoo-kept Bactrian camels, Père David's deer, and gnus.[41–44] Ruminants appear to have reduced sensitivity to HGA, possibly due to differences in HGA metabolism.[45] The first step of conversion of HGA to its toxic metabolite is catalysis by BCAA aminotransferase, which has lower activity in skeletal muscle of ruminants compared to monogastric species.[46] Ruminal degradation of HGA, especially in species with longer ruminal retention time of solutes, may be another reason for decreased susceptibility to HGA poisoning.[44]

Other sources of hypoglycin A

In addition to *Acer* species, HGA has also been documented in fruits from other trees of the Sapindaceae family, including ackee (*Blighia sapida*) and litchi (*Litchi chinensis*).[47] Human consumption of unripe ackee fruit causes Jamaican vomiting disease, while ingestion of litchi fruit, which also contains MCPG, has been linked to cases of acute hypoglycemic encephalopathy.[48,49] In contrast to myopathy and hyperglycemia observed in horses, HGA poisoning in humans appears to primarily affect the liver and the clinical picture is dominated by severe, often fatal hypoglycemia.

WHITE SNAKEROOT AND RAYLESS GOLDENROD—INTRODUCTION/BACKGROUND
Plant Names and Descriptions

White snakeroot (*Ageratina altissima,* formerly *E rugosum*) and rayless goldenrod (*I pluriflora*, formerly *Haplopappus heterophyllus*) are up to 1.5-m-tall perennial herbs belonging to the family Asteraceae (the aster family). White snakeroot is predominantly found in the eastern half of North America in moist, partially shaded areas such as woodlands, thickets, stream banks, and terraces.[50] It has sharply serrated simple leaves and blooms from late summer to fall, displaying clusters of small, white, composite flowers (**Fig. 2A–C**). Rayless goldenrod inhabits the Southwestern United States and Northern Mexico, preferentially growing in alkaline, calcareous soil. It is commonly found on dry rangelands in Arizona, Colorado, New Mexico, and Texas. Rayless goldenrod forms unbranched, erect, woody stems, with alternate, narrow leaves, crowned by a cluster of golden-yellow flowers that bloom from spring to fall (**Fig. 3A–C**).

Associated Toxidromes and Suspected Toxic Principles

Following naturally occurring and/or experimental ingestion of toxic amounts, both plants can cause a similar disease process in horses, characterized by nonexertional rhabdomyolysis and cardiac myonecrosis. White snakeroot has historical significance as the cause of "milk sickness," a condition arising from consumption of milk from cows consuming white snakeroot. "Milk sickness" led to the death of many settlers, including, reportedly, Abraham Lincoln's mother, in the Midwestern United States in

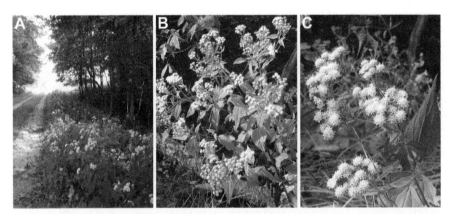

Fig. 2. Multiple white snakeroot (*Ageratina altissima*) plants are shown growing near a wooded area during the fall (*A*). (*B*) shows an individual white snakeroot (*A altissima*) plant growing near a stream in a wooded area during the fall, and (*C*) shows the characteristic small white flowers and typical leaves of white snakeroot (*A altissima*) in greater detail. (Image courtesy [*A*] Dr. T. Zane Davis, USDA Poisonous Plant Research Laboratory in Logan, Utah; and [*B* and *C*] Dr. Tim Evans, University of Missouri-Columbia.)

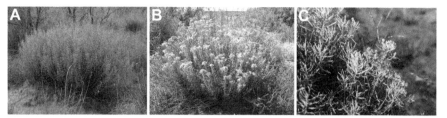

Fig. 3. A rayless goldenrod (*Isocoma pluriflora*) plant without inflorescence is shown in (*A*). (*B*) shows a rayless goldenrod (*I pluriflora*) plant with flowers and (*C*) shows the characteristic flowers of rayless goldenrod (*I pluriflora*). (Image courtesy [*A* and *C*] Dr. T. Zane Davis, USDA Poisonous Plant Research Laboratory in Logan, Utah; and [*B*] Dr. Samantha Uhrig, Carlsbad, New Mexico.)

the early 19th century. In cattle, white snakeroot poisoning causes progressive muscular weakness and tremors, known as "trembles." By 1930, a compound referred to as "tremetol" was identified as the toxic component in both white snakeroot and rayless goldenrod.[51,52] "Tremetol" was later discovered to be a complex mixture of benzofuran ketones (BFKs), including tremetone, dehydrotremetone, hydroxytremetone, and oxy-angeloyltremetone (**Fig. 4**A and B).[53,54] Additionally, diverse phenols and chromenes have also been isolated from white snakeroot.[55,56] The individual, additive, and/or synergistic roles these compounds may play in the toxicity of white snakeroot and rayless goldenrod remain unknown. Tremetone had long been considered the major toxin in the "tremetol" mixture and has proven concentration-dependent cytotoxic effects in vitro.[57] However, in contrast to "tremetol," purified tremetone elicited no signs of

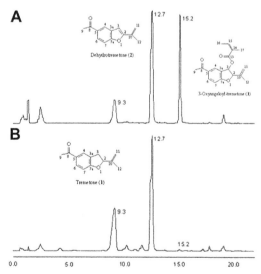

Fig. 4. The structures of 3 major benzofuran ketone compounds associated with rayless goldenrod (*Isocoma pluriflora*) and/or white snakeroot (*Ageratina altissima*) are shown along with their high-performance liquid chromatography (HPLC) chromatograms in (*A*) and (*B*), respectively. Note that tremetone appears to be present in greater concentrations in white snakeroot than in rayless goldenrod, and, conversely, 3-oxyangeloyltremetone appears to be present only in rayless goldenrod. (Images courtesy Dr. Stephen T. Lee, USDA Poisonous Plant Research Laboratory in Logan, Utah.)

toxicosis in chickens.[58] Quantification of tremetone, dehydrotremetone, and 3-oxyan-geloyl-tremetone in white snakeroot and rayless goldenrod via high-performance liquid chromatography, as shown in **Fig. 4**A and B, revealed great variability in BFK content between different collections of both plant species.[54] Furthermore, white snakeroot plants collected from different Midwestern states showed not only chemical but also toxicologic variation, with some samples apparently not being "toxic." There appeared to be no direct correlation between relative plant toxicity in goats and plant tremetone and total BFK content.[56] Similarly, tremetone content did not correlate with severity of clinical signs in calves with experimental rayless goldenrod (and goldenbush, *I acradenia*) toxicosis.[59] Collectively, these findings put the toxic potential of tremetone further into question, at least in poultry and ruminants, and suggests the possibility of a previously unidentified toxic metabolite, an entirely new toxin, and/or, possibly, complex synergistic interactions between individual BFKs, which are ultimately responsible for the observed clinical signs of intoxication. However, these experimental results involving primarily ruminants do not necessarily definitively rule out the role of tremetone and its various metabolites in causing white snakeroot intoxication in horses.

Toxic Mechanisms of Action

Not surprisingly for a complex mixture, "tremetol's" toxic mechanism of action is not well understood. Wu *and colleagues* reported a drastic inhibition of mitochondrial citrate synthase, the enzyme catalyzing the first step in the Krebs cycle, and decreased glucose utilization following intramuscular injections of "tremetol" in chickens.[60] This suggests that disruption of oxidative cellular energy metabolism plays a role in the clinical manifestation of the toxicosis. Tremetone may require hepatic metabolism to unfold its toxic activity and likely undergoes enterohepatic recycling resulting in cumulative effects.[61,62] Excretion of "tremetol" and its constituent BFKs in the milk may act as a route of detoxification, but the presence of these toxins in the milk poses a risk to suckling foals.[63]

CLINICAL ASPECTS OF WHITE SNAKEROOT/RAYLESS GOLDENROD INTOXICATIONS IN HORSES
Incidence

White snakeroot poisoning in horses generally only occurs sporadically in the United States, in part, due to differences in chemical composition and toxic potential of ingested plants. Susceptibility of individual animals may also vary depending on their nutritional status and antioxidant potential.[56,64] In fact, one of the authors observed a suspected case of white snakeroot intoxication involving a previously obese horse, which after being deprived of any feedstuffs other than what was growing in its small pen, including white snakeroot plants eventually stripped of most of their foliage and inflorescence, had lost a significant amount of weight prior to the onset of clinical signs characteristic of white snakeroot intoxication. It is likely that the rapidly induced loss of adipose tissue in this animal enhanced the bioavailability of the BFKs to which it was exposed. Naturally occurring rayless goldenrod poisoning has not been reported in horses, but the toxic principles, clinical presentation, and postmortem findings of experimentally induced intoxication closely resemble those of white snakeroot toxicosis. In this experimental setting, horses developed signs of toxicity following daily ingestion of rayless goldenrod at 1.5% and 3% of bodyweight (BW), containing 30 and 60 mg BFK/kg BW, over a period of 10 to 14 days.[57]

Clinical Signs of White Snakeroot Intoxication in Horses

Horses seem to be particularly susceptible to the toxic effects of white snakeroot and may die within 1 to 2 days after onset of clinical signs. Cardiac involvement is substantial and is accompanied by varying degrees of nonexertional rhabdomyolysis. Common clinical signs include depression, tachycardia, arrhythmia, profuse sweating, muscular weakness, reluctance to move, stiffness, prolonged recumbency, and myoglobinuria. Muscle tremors are not as consistent or as severe, compared to cattle.[50] Dyspnea, dysphagia, esophageal obstruction, and decreased fecal output have also been reported.[63,65,66] Ventral edema and circulatory compromise may develop due to congestive heart failure.[62]

Diagnosis

Antemortem diagnosis
Elevations in muscle enzyme activities (CK, AST) and cardiac troponin I concentrations correlate with the degree of skeletal and cardiac myonecrosis. Increased concentrations of cardiac troponin I may be a sensitive early indicator of toxicity. Electrocardiographic changes include premature ventricular contractions, atrioventricular block, and ST segment depression.[62] Urinalysis may show myoglobinuria. Detection of tremetone and other BFKs in biological samples from affected animals (ie, urine, blood, serum) confirms a diagnosis of white snakeroot intoxication and, likewise, would be critical for the documentation of naturally occurring rayless goldenrod intoxication in a horse. However, analyses for these compounds are not currently available in many veterinary diagnostic laboratories.

Postmortem diagnosis
Postmortem evaluation reveals swelling, pallor, and occasional streaking of the large appendicular skeletal muscles (especially quadriceps femoris and superficial pectoral) and myocardium. In contrast to other animal species, lesions in the cardiac muscle are typically reported to be more prominent than pathologic changes in the skeletal muscle of horses. In equine species, there is usually histopathologic evidence of severe myofiber degeneration and necrosis, as well as evidence of mineralization and fibrosis.[50,57] Hepatic congestion with centrilobular fatty changes and renal tubular necrosis and mineralization have also been reported in horses.[62] As with antemortem diagnosis of white snakeroot intoxication in horses, analyses for BFKs are not readily available in many veterinary diagnostic laboratories; however, detection of these compounds in postmortem biological samples (ie, aqueous humor, stomach contents, liver, and kidney) confirms a diagnosis of white snakeroot or, potentially, rayless goldenrod intoxication.

Differential Diagnoses

With respect to any observed rhabdomyolysis, the differential diagnoses for white snakeroot intoxication and possible rayless goldenrod intoxication would include SPM/AM and the wide range of differential diagnoses listed for those diseases.[23] With respect to myocardial necrosis, which appears to be a predominant feature of intoxications involving white snakeroot (and presumably also *Isocoma* species), differential diagnoses include exposures to cantharidin in blister beetle–contaminated alfalfa hay; concentrates or supplements containing ionophores, especially monensin; prolonged exposures to cardiotoxic plants, such as yew (*Taxus* species) and cardiac glycoside–containing plants, including oleander (*Nerium oleander*), milkweeds (*Asclepias* species), hemp dogbane (*Apocynum cannabinum*), as well as other plant species; and exposures to other toxicants associated with myocardial necrosis and heart failure.[67]

TREATMENT

Treatment of horses with white snakeroot intoxication and, presumably, rayless goldenrod poisoning is symptomatic and should include supportive care such as IV fluids to correct any electrolyte or acid-base derangements, maintain perfusion, and provide diuresis to prevent pigment nephropathy. Analgesics may be indicated to control pain associated with myonecrosis.[67] Antioxidants (vitamin C, vitamin E/selenium) may help prevent oxidative damage associated with impaired cellular energy metabolism. If significant arrhythmias are present, administration of antiarrhythmic drugs is indicated.[67] Oral administration of charcoal may reduce intestinal absorption and decrease enterohepatic recycling of the toxin. This can be accompanied by a single dose of a laxative to hasten intestinal transit time of the toxin. Administration of charcoal and a laxative may also serve as a preventative measure in other horses in the same pasture, which may have also been exposed but are currently subclinical. Additionally, restricting movement and decreasing stress may help prevent exacerbation of clinical signs in affected horses or precipitation of clinical signs in exposed horses.[68] The prognosis for white snakeroot intoxication in horses and, presumably, rayless goldenrod intoxication is generally poor, although mildly affected animals, without obvious cardiac involvement, may fully recover within 2 weeks. More severely affected horses may take several weeks to recover and may experience late complications in the form of congestive heart failure.[67]

PREVENTION

The best preventative measure is to prohibit horses from having access to areas of pastures and/or woodlands where white snakeroot is growing. While naturally occurring rayless goldenrod intoxication is yet to be diagnosed, intentionally grazing horses in areas where this plant commonly grows would be considered inadvisable, especially when limited forage is available for consumption. The risk of white snakeroot intoxication is expected to be higher in the fall, when this plant is most prevalent, and this increased risk is especially heightened during years when pastures contain little in the way of grass and horses browse for additional feedstuffs. Since BFKs have been reported to remain active after freezing, the risk of intoxication persists through winter.[62,68,69] Furthermore, there is reportedly little reduction in toxic potential after drying of white snakeroot and rayless goldenrod, resulting in hay contaminated with these plants being another potential source of their toxins.[70]

While naturally occurring instances of rayless goldenrod poisoning in horses have yet to be documented, this apparent rarity of equine intoxications involving *I pluriflora* does not rule out the potential toxicity of other *Isocoma* species. Recent research documented the presence of tremetone and other BFKs in diverse *Isocoma* species found in the Southwestern United States, and, subsequently, calves fed goldenbush (*I acradenia*) developed clinical signs very similar to those of rayless goldenrod toxicosis.[59,71]

SUMMARY

Boxelder and sycamore maple seeds and seedlings contain HGA, the toxic metabolite of which, MCPA-CoA, inhibits fatty acid β-oxidation, causing SPM and AM in the United States and Europe, respectively. White snakeroot and rayless goldenrod contain BFKs, the identity and toxicity of which appear somewhat variable and possibly dependent on complex interactions between these compounds. BFKs as well as their metabolites also appear to inhibit cellular energy metabolism. While skeletal and cardiac muscle are both susceptible to the toxic effects of all these toxins, SPM/AM involves predominantly postural and respiratory muscles, and cardiac myonecrosis is more consistent and pronounced in white snakeroot intoxication. Animals in poor body condition, especially those grazing on pastures with sparse vegetation during the fall, appear to be predisposed to developing these plant-associated conditions. The toxins in these plants remain toxic in hay and are excreted in milk. Management of these frequently fatal toxidromes focuses on plant identification, early diagnosis, supportive treatment, and, ideally, prevention.

CLINICS CARE POINTS

- Plant-induced toxic myopathies are most common in the fall and are frequently fatal.
- Animals in poor body condition, especially those grazing on pastures with sparse vegetation, are predisposed.
- Hay containing these toxic plants and milk from mares exposed to these plants can serve as sources of intoxication.
- SPM/AM affects predominantly postural and respiratory muscles, while white snakeroot intoxication results in more pronounced cardiac myonecrosis.
- Dyspnea, dysphagia, esophageal obstruction and signs of colic are common and may mimic other disease processes.
- Serum muscle enzyme activities and cardiac troponin I are typically markedly elevated and serve as useful diagnostic tests.
- No specific antidote is available and treatment is supportive, including analgesic, antioxidant and IV fluid therapy.
- Immediate referral to a tertiary care facility, especially early in the course of these intoxications, may improve prognosis for survival.
- Exposed, subclinical co-grazers should be monitored closely to ensure early diagnosis.

DISCLOSURES

The authors have no disclosures.

REFERENCES

1. USDA, NRCS. *Acer negundo* L. Plant Profile. In: The PLANTS Database; National Plant Data Team, Greensboro, NC USA. Available at: http://plants.usda.gov. Accessed June 7, 2023.
2. Pasta S, de Rigo D, Caudullo G. *Acer pseudoplatanus* in Europe: distribution, habitat, usage and threats. In: San-Miguel-Ayanz J, de Rigo D, Caudullo G, et al, editors. European atlas of forest tree species. Luxembourg: Publication Office of the European Union; 2016. p. 56–8.
3. USDA, NRCS. Boxelder, *Acer negundo* L. Plant Guide. In: The PLANTS Database; National Plant Data Team, Greensboro, NC USA. Available at: http://plants.usda.gov. Accessed June 7, 2023.
4. Valberg SJ, Sponseller BT, Hegeman AD, et al. Seasonal pasture myopathy/atypical myopathy in North America associated with ingestion of hypoglycin A within seeds of the box elder tree. Equine Vet J 2013;45:419–25.
5. Votion DM, van Galen G, Sweetman L, et al. Identification of methylenecyclopropyl acetic acid in serum of European horses with atypical myopathy. Equine Vet J 2014;46:146–9.
6. Unger L, Nicholson A, Jewitt EM, et al. Hypoglycin concentrations in seeds of *Acer pseudoplatanus* trees growing on atypical myopathy-affected and control pastures. J Vet Intern Med 2014;28:1289–93.

7. Kean ER. Hypoglycin. In: Cheeke PR, editor. Toxicants of plant origin. Boca Raton, FL: CRC Press; 1989. p. 229–62.

8. Ikeda Y, Tanaka K. Selective inactivation of various acyl-CoA dehydrogenases by (methylenecyclopropyl)acetyl-CoA. Biochim Biophys Acta 1990;1038:216–21.

9. Bochnia M, Sander J, Ziegler J, et al. Detection of MCPG metabolites in horses with atypical myopathy. PLoS One 2019;14(2):e0211698.

10. Sander J, Terhardt M, Sander S, et al. A new method for quantifying causative and diagnostic markers of methylenecyclopropylglycine poisoning. Toxicol Rep 2019;6:803–8.

11. Li D, Agnihotri G, Dakoji S, et al. The toxicity of methylenecyclopropylglycine: studies of the inhibitory effects of (methylenecyclopropyl)formyl-CoA on enzymes involved in fatty acid metabolism and the molecular basis of its inactivation of Enoyl-CoA hydratases. J Am Chem Soc 1999;121:3034–42.

12. Van Galen G, Marcillaud PC, Saegerman C, et al. European outbreaks of atypical myopathy in grazing equids (2006-2009): spatiotemporal distribution, history and clinical features. Equine Vet J 2012;44:614–20.

13. Sponseller BT, Valberg SJ, Schultz NE, et al. Equine multiple acyl-CoA dehydrogenase deficiency (MADD) associated with seasonal pasture myopathy in the Midwestern United States. J Vet Intern Med 2012;26:1012–8.

14. Votion DM, Linden A, Saegerman C. History and clinical features of atypical myopathy in horses in Belgium (2000-2005). J Vet Intern Med 2007;21:1380–91.

15. Verheyen T, Decloedt A, De Clercq D, et al. Cardiac changes in horses with atypical myopathy. J Vet Intern Med 2012;26:1019–26.

16. Westermann CM, Dorland L, Votion DM, et al. Acquired multiple acyl-CoA dehydrogenase deficiency in 10 horses with atypical myopathy. Neuromuscul Disord 2008;18:355–64.

17. Sander J, Terhardt M, Sander S, et al. Use of a standard newborn screening test for the rapid diagnosis of inhibited ß-oxidation in atypical myopathy in horses. J Equine Vet Sci 2018;67:71–4.

18. Boemer F, Detilleux J, Cello C, et al. Acylcarnitines profile best predicts survival in horses with atypical myopathy. PLoS One 2017;12(8):e0182761.

19. González-Medina S, Hyde C, Lovera I, et al. Detection of hypoglycin A and MCPA-carnitine in equine serum and muscle tissue: Optimisation and validation of a LC-MS-based method without derivatization. Equine Vet J 2021;53:558–68.

20. Sander J, Cavalleri J-MV, Terhardt M, et al. Rapid diagnosis of hypoglycin A intoxication in atypical myopathy of horses. J Vet Diagn Invest 2016;28:98–104.

21. Finno CS, Valberg SJ, Wünschmann A, et al. Seasonal pasture myopathy in horses in the midwestern United States: 14 cases (1998-2005). J Am Vet Med Assoc 2006;229:1134–41.

22. Votion DM, Serteyn D. Equine atypical myopathy: A review. Vet J 2008;178:185–90.

23. Votion DM. The story of equine atypical myopathy: A review from the beginning to a possible end. ISRN Vet Sci 2012;2012:281018.

24. Westermann CM, van Leeuwen R, van Raamsdonk LWD, et al. Hypoglycin A concentrations in maple tree species in the Netherlands and the occurrence of atypical myopathy in horses. J Vet Intern Med 2016;30:880–4.

25. Bowen-Forbes CS, Minott DA. Tracking hypoglycins A and B over different maturity stages: implications for detoxification of ackee (Blighia sapida K.D. Koenig) fruits. J Agric Food Chem 2011;59:3869–75.

26. González-Medina S, Hyde C, Lovera I, et al. Detection of equine atypical myopathy-associated hypoglycin A in plant material: Optimisation and validation

of a novel LC-MS based method without derivatization. PLoS One 2018;13(7): e0199521.

27. El-Khatib AH, Engel AM, Weigel S. Co-occurrence of hypoglycin A and hypoglycin B in sycamore and box elder maple proved by LC-MS/MS and LC-HR-MS. Toxins 2022;14:608.

28. van Galen G, Votion DM. Management of cases suffering from atypical myopathy: Interpretations of descriptive, epidemiological and pathophysiological findings. Part 2: Muscular, urinary, respiratory and hepatic care, and inflammatory/infectious status. Equine Vet Educ 2013;25:264–70.

29. Hovda TK. Boxelder (*Acer negundo*). In: Hovda LR, Benson D, Poppenga RH, editors. *Blackwell's five-minute veterinary consult clinical companion: equine toxicology*. 1st edition. Hoboken, NJ: John Wiley & Sons; 2021. p. 437–41. https://doi. org/10.1002/9781119671527.ch83.

30. Fabius LS, Westermann CM. Evidence-based therapy for atypical myopathy in horses. Equine Vet Educ 2018;30:616–22.

31. El-Gharbawy A, Vockley J. Defects of fatty acid oxidation and the carnitine shuttle system. Pediatr Clin North Am 2018;65:317–35.

32. Krägeloh T, Cavalleri JMV, Ziegler J, et al. Identification of hypoglycin A binding adsorbents as potential preventative measures in co-grazers of atypical myopathy affected horses. Equine Vet J 2018;50:220–7.

33. Bochnia M, Ziegler J, Sander J, et al. Hypoglycin A content in blood and urine discriminates horses with atypical myopathy from clinically normal horses grazing on the same pasture. PLoS One 2015;10(9):e0136785.

34. Wouters CP, Toquet MP, Renaud B, et al. Metabolomic signatures discriminate horses with clinical signs of atypical myopathy from healthy co-grazing horses. J Proteome Res 2021;20:4681–92.

35. Votion DM, Habyarimana JA, Scippo ML, et al. Potential new sources of hypoglycin A poisoning for equids kept at pasture in spring: a field pilot study. Vet Rec 2019;184:740.

36. González-Medina S, Montesso F, Chang Y-M, et al. Atypical myopathy-associated hypoglycin A toxin remains in sycamore seedlings despite mowing, herbicidal spraying or storage in hay and silage. Equine Vet J 2019;51:701–4.

37. Karlíková R, Široká J, Mech M, et al. Newborn foal with atypical myopathy. J Vet Intern Med 2018;32:1768–72.

38. Sander J, Terhardt M, Janzen N. Detection of maple toxins in mare's milk. J Vet Intern Med 2021;35:606–9.

39. Renaud B, François AC, Boemer F, et al. Grazing mares on pasture with sycamore maples: A potential threat to suckling foals and food safety through milk contamination. Animals 2021;11:87.

40. Bochnia M, Ziegler J, Glatter M, et al. Hypoglycin A in Cow's Milk—A Pilot Study. Toxins 2021;13:381.

41. Hirz M, Gregersen HA, Sander J, et al. Atypical myopathy in 2 Bactrian camels. J Vet Diagn Invest 2021;33:961–5.

42. Bunert C, Langer, Votion DM, et al. Atypical myopathy in Père David's deer (*Elaphurus davidianus*) associated with ingestion of hypoglycin A. J Anim Sci 2018; 96:3537–47.

43. Bochnia M, Ziemssen E, Sander J, et al. Methylenecyclopropylglycine and hypoglycin A intoxication in three Père David's Deer (*Elaphurus davidianus*) with atypical myopathy. Vet Med Sci 2021;7:998–1005.

44. Renaud B, Kruse CJ, François AC, et al. *Acer pseudoplatanus*: A potential risk of poisoning for several herbivore species. Toxins 2022;14:512.

45. González-Medina S, Bevin W, Alzola-Domingo R, et al. Hypoglycin A absorption in sheep without concurrent clinical or biochemical evidence of disease. J Vet Intern Med 2021;35:1170–6.
46. Papet I, Grizard J, Bonin D, et al. Regulation of branched chain amino acid metabolism in ruminants. Diabete Metab 1992;18:122–8.
47. Sanford AA, Isenberg SL, Carter MD, et al. Quantitative HPLC–MS/MS analysis of toxins in soapberry seeds: Methylenecyclopropylglycine and hypoglycin A. Food Chem 2018;264:449–54.
48. Joskow R, Belson M, Vesper H, et al. Ackee fruit poisoning: an outbreak investigation in Haiti 2000-2001, and review of the literature. Clin Toxicol 2006;44: 267–73.
49. Shrivastava A, Kumar A, Thomas JD, et al. Association of acute toxic encephalopathy with litchi consumption in an outbreak in Muzaffarpur, India, 2014: a case control study. Lancet Global Health 2017;5:e458–66.
50. Burrows GE, Tyrl RJ. Asteraceae Martinov. In: Burrows GE, Tyrl RJ, editors. Toxic plants of North America. 2nd edition. Hoboken, NJ: Wiley-Blackwell; 2012. p. 150–256. https://doi.org/10.1002/9781118413425.ch13.
51. Couch JF. The toxic constituent of richweed or white snakeroot (Eupatorium urticaefolium). J Agric Res 1927;35:547–76.
52. Couch JF. The toxic constituent of rayless goldenrod. J Agric Res 1930;40: 649–58.
53. Bonner WA, De Graw JI, Bowen DM, et al. Toxic constituents of white snakeroot. Tetrahedron Lett 1961;12:417–20.
54. Lee AT, Davis TZ, Gardner DR, et al. Quantitative method for the measurement of three benzofuran ketones in rayless goldenrod (Isocoma pluriflora) and white snake root (Ageratina altissima) by High-Performance Liquid Chromatography (HPLC). J Agric Food Chem 2009;57:5639–43.
55. Lee ST, Davis TZ, Gardner DR, et al. Tremetone and structurally related compounds in white snakeroot (Ageratina altissima): A plant associated with trembles and milk sickness. J Agric Food Chem 2010;58:8560–5.
56. Davis TZ, Stegelmeier BL, Lee ST, et al. White snakeroot poisoning in goats: Variations in toxicity with different plant chemotypes. Res Vet Sci 2016;106:29–36.
57. Davis TZ, Stegelmeier BL, Lee ST, et al. Experimental rayless goldenrod (Isocoma pluriflora) toxicosis in horses. Toxicon 2013;73:88–95.
58. Bowen DM, DeGraw JI, Shah VR, et al. The synthesis and pharmacological action of tremetone. J Med Chem 1963;6:315–9.
59. Davis TZ, Green BT, Stegelmeier BL. The comparative toxicity of Isocoma species in calves. Toxicon X 2020;5.
60. Wu CH, Lampe KF, Mende TJ. Metabolic changes induced in chickens by the administration of tremetol. Biochem Pharmacol 1973;22:2835–41.
61. Beier RC, Norman JO, Reagor JC, et al. Isolation of the major component in white snakeroot that is toxic after microsomal activation: Possible explanation of sporadic toxicity of white snakeroot plants and extracts. Nat Toxins 1993;1:286–93.
62. Smetzer DL, Coppock RW, Ely RW, et al. Cardiac effects of white snakeroot intoxication in horses. Equine Pract 1983;5:26–32.
63. Sanders M. White snakeroot poisoning in a foal: a case report. J Equine Vet Sci 1983;3:128–31.
64. Stegelmeier BL, Davis TZ, Green BT, et al. Experimental rayless goldenrod (Isocoma pluriflora) toxicosis in goats. J Vet Diagn Invest 2010;22:570–7.
65. Olson CT, Keller WC, Gerken DF, et al. Suspected tremetol poisoning in horses. J Am Vet Med Assoc 1984;185:1001–3.

66. Thompson LJ. Depression and choke in a horse: probable white snakeroot toxicosis. Vet Hum Toxicol 1989;31:321–2.
67. Ward CM. White Snakeroot (*Ageratina altissima*). In: Hovda LR, Benson D, Poppenga RH, editors. Blackwell's five-minute veterinary consult clinical companion: equine toxicology. 1st edition. Hoboken, NJ: John Wiley & Sons; 2021. p. 364–8. https://doi.org/10.1002/9781119671527.ch70.
68. Barr AC, Reagor JC. Toxic plants: What the horse practitioner needs to know. Vet Clin N Am Equine Pract 2001;17:529–46.
69. Lee ST, Davis TZ, Cook D. Evaluation of the stability of benzofuran ketones in rayless goldenrod (Isocoma pluriflora) and white snakeroot (*Ageratina altissima*) under different storage conditions. In: International Journal of Poisonous Plant Research. 2017. Available at: https://www.ars.usda.gov/ARSUserFiles/oc/np/PoisonousPlants/Fall2017/goldenrod.pdf. Accessed August 4, 2023.
70. Lee ST, Davis TZ, Cook D, et al. Evaluation of drying methods and toxicity of rayless goldenrod (*Isocoma pluriflora*) and white snakeroot (*Ageratina altissima*) in goats. J Agric Food Chem 2012;60:4849–53.
71. Lee ST, Cook D, Davis TZ, et al. A survey of tremetone, dehydrotremetone, and structurally related compounds in *Isocoma* spp. (goldenbush) in the Southwestern United States. J Agric Food Chem 2015;63:872–9.

Toxic Garden and Landscaping Plants

Megan C. Romano, DVM

KEYWORDS

- Poisonous • Toxic • Plants • Yew • *Taxus* • Oleander • *Nerium* • Equine

KEY POINTS

- Horses are most often exposed to toxic garden and landscaping plants when trimmings or clippings are discarded within reach or contaminate hay.
- Treatment of toxic plant ingestion in horses can be unrewarding due to its acute, rapidly progressive nature, so client education aimed at prevention is critical.
- Activated charcoal with or without cathartics may be useful in recent toxic plant ingestions in horses.
- Antidotes are either unavailable or prohibitively expensive for most toxic plant ingestions in horses; treatment is primarily symptomatic and supportive.

INTRODUCTION

The medicinal and toxic properties of many plants have been known for centuries. Bark, berries, and leaves of such plants have been used as early folk remedies, fish poisons, hunting aids, "ordeal poisons," and murder weapons. Teas, tinctures, and tablets developed from plants formed the basis of early pharmacopeias.[1] Plant poisonings have been well documented in humans and animals due to accidental or intentional exposures.

Horses and other equines can be exposed to toxic plants in pastures or on rangelands, via contaminated hay or grain, and through gardening and landscaping activity. Tree trimmings, storm-downed limbs, lawn clippings, and fallen leaves can end up within reach of hungry or curious animals, or can be intentionally fed by well-meaning owners or neighbors who are ignorant of the danger. Preventive measures include keeping the plants, including trimmings and leaves, out of reach of animals, educating neighbors to do the same, and purchasing weed-free hay from reputable suppliers.

The following are some of the most common garden and landscaping plants in North America that can be toxic to equines when ingested in sufficient quantities.

Department of Veterinary Science, Veterinary Diagnostic Laboratory, University of Kentucky, 1490 Bull Lea Road, PO Box 14125, Lexington, KY 40512-4125, USA
E-mail address: megan.romano@uky.edu

Vet Clin Equine 40 (2024) 61–76
https://doi.org/10.1016/j.cveq.2023.11.002
0749-0739/24/© 2023 Elsevier Inc. All rights reserved.

Plants and their ranges are briefly described; additional, regularly updated information and plant distribution maps are available at the United States Department of Agriculture's Plant List of Attributes, Names, Taxonomy, and Symbols (USDA PLANTS) database https://plants.usda.gov/home.

YEW (*TAXUS SPP.*)

Yew trees (*Taxus* spp) have been associated with the magical and mystical since antiquity; their well-known toxic properties led to the nickname "Tree of Death." Yew remains toxic when dried, and poisoning in livestock is often due to discarded plant clippings being placed within the reach of curious animals.[2,3] Some species seem relatively palatable, especially when mixed with lawn clippings. Bored or stressed horses are most likely to eat yew clippings.[2]

Yew is a low-maintenance evergreen shrub or tree, and yew hedges are popular landscaping plants in many parts of North America.[4] North American species include the native *Taxus brevifolia* Nutt. (western or Pacific yew), *Taxus canadensis* Marshall (Canada or American yew or ground hemlock), and *Taxus floridana* Nutt. ex Chapm. (Florida yew), and the introduced *Taxus baccata* L. (English yew), *Taxus cuspidata* Siebold & Zucc (Japanese yew), and *Taxus* ×*media* Rehder [*baccata* × *cuspidata*] (hybrid yew).[4]

Taxus leaves are simple, alternate, and flat or needlelike.[4] Mature leaves are approximately 0.5 to 1 inch long, dark green, glossy, and stiff, with a prominent midrib and a sharp, pointed tip (**Fig. 1**A–C). Young leaves are softer and lighter green. The nutlike seeds are partially enclosed in a bright red, berrylike aril.

All parts of the plant except for the aril contain volatile irritant oils and cardiotoxic taxine alkaloids.[4] Variability in concentrations of irritant oils likely causes the variation in palatability between yew species. Cardiotoxic effects are due to taxines, primarily taxine B, concentrations of which can also vary among species.[5]

Mechanism

Taxines are cardioselective calcium and sodium channel antagonists.[5] Altered calcium and sodium conductance results in increased cytoplasmic calcium and dose-dependent inhibition of calcium-induced contractions. Atrio-ventricular (AV)

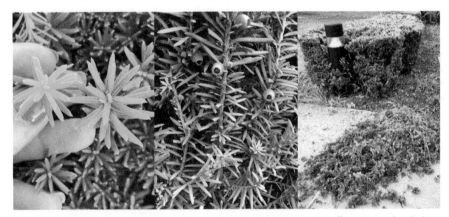

Fig. 1. Yew (*Taxus* spp). Immature (L) and mature (R) leaves/needles. Note the lighter, brighter green of the immature leaves (*A*). Berries (arils) with seeds inside, leaves (*B*). Pile of yew clippings after landscaping (*C*).

conduction abnormalities can result in a second-degree or third-degree AV block or complete heart block (diastolic asystole).[5]

Toxic Dose

Horses seem more sensitive than other species to taxines.[5] Approximately 0.1% body weight of green *T cuspidata* foliage and berries administered to a Shetland Pony mare was lethal.[6]

Clinical Signs, Examination Findings, and Laboratory Confirmation

Often, the sudden death of a previously healthy animal is the only finding with yew poisoning. Horses and donkeys have collapsed and died with no signs of struggling or convulsions within minutes of ingestion.[2] In the Shetland Pony mare, lip and tail paresis developed within 1 hour.[6] The pony developed ataxia, muscle tremors, and respiratory grunting before collapsing into lateral recumbency. Death occurred within 15 minutes of onset of signs. Other reported signs in horses with yew poisoning include weakness and tremors, abdominal pain, dyspnea, convulsions, and rapid death.[7]

Postmortem findings in peracute cases are often nonspecific. Pulmonary congestion and hemorrhage or edema; hepatic and splenic congestion; hemorrhagic pericardial effusion; endocardial hemorrhage; hemorrhage and edema of gastrointestinal (GI) serosa and mucosa; and identifiable plant material in the GI tract have been reported.[7–9]

Animals that survive long enough may develop cardiac lesions including acute multifocal contraction band necrosis.[7] Yew leaves may be observed in the mouth, esophagus, or stomach.[2,7] Some diagnostic laboratories can also analyze GI contents or plant material for taxine alkaloids or their metabolites.[10]

Treatment

Because of the rapid onset and progression of clinical signs, treatment is rarely possible. Affected animals should be kept quiet, and stress and activity minimized. For recent ingestions, gastric lavage via nasogastric (NG) tube followed by instillation of activated charcoal (AC) and cathartics can be considered.[4] Patients that survive acute intoxication often require symptomatic and supportive care and can suffer fatal arrhythmias after apparently recovering. Calves that initially survived yew poisoning died suddenly several days afterward with lesions including myocardial fibrosis.[11]

OLEANDER AND OTHER CARDIAC GLYCOSIDE-CONTAINING PLANTS

Cardioactive glycosides (cardiac glycosides) are produced by certain plants to discourage herbivory. Foxglove (*Digitalis spp.*), with its instantly recognizable spikes of bell-shaped flowers, is probably the most famous and the most infamous. Herbal remedies and purified *Digitalis* glycosides have been used for centuries as cardiac tonics, diuretics, and emetics.[12] More recently, cardiac glycosides have been investigated as chemotherapeutic agents.[13]

Cardiac glycosides are considered poorly water soluble; however, animals have been poisoned by drinking water into which oleander leaves have fallen, and humans have been poisoned by soups stirred with oleander branches.[14] Although most fresh green plants seem unpalatable, toxicity is retained after drying. Cases have occurred when tree or shrub trimmings are left within reach or unintentionally mixed with lawn clippings or hay, or when animals ingest fallen leaves.[14–16]

Mechanism

Cardiac glycosides inhibit plasma membrane sodium-potassium pumps (Na^+/K^+-ATPases).[17] Na^+/K^+-ATPases maintain Na^+ and K^+ concentration gradients and electrostatic potential (electrochemical gradients) across cell membranes.[18] Electrochemical gradients are essential for action potential propagation in cardiomyocytes and other excitable cells; inhibition of Na^+/K^+-ATPase causes elevated intracellular sodium concentration and disrupts the electrochemical gradient.[18] Elevated sodium concentrations also inhibit sodium-calcium (Na^+-Ca^{2+}) channels, causing elevated intracellular calcium. Cardiomyocytes are particularly sensitive to elevated intracellular calcium; conduction abnormalities and ventricular arrhythmias can result.[19] The positive inotropic and negative chronotropic actions can be beneficial in certain kinds of cardiac disease; however, in excessive doses altered cardiac conduction can result in arrhythmias. At toxic doses, other excitable cells (eg, neurons, GI smooth muscle, and skeletal muscle) can also be affected.

Toxic Dose

The toxicity of cardiac glycoside-containing plants can vary widely depending on plant and animal type. Plant factors include species and chemotype. Animal factors include species, age, health status, comorbidities, coingestion of other toxicants, and a variety of other factors. For example, in one report, 4 of 6 horses fed hay contaminated with 8.5% *Adonis aestivalis* died, whereas the remaining 2 horses only developed diarrhea.[20]

In a series of oleander administration studies, an estimated minimum toxic dose was approximately 10 g green leaves in an adult horse (20 mg/kg; 0.002% body weight) (**Table 1**).[14] Ten (10) g green leaves administered in a bran mash to an adult mare produced "no perceptible change" but an adult gelding administered an aqueous infusion made from 10 g green leaves developed diarrhea after 24 h. Doses of 25 g green leaves (50 mg/kg; 0.005% body weight) and 14 g dry leaves (30 mg/kg; 0.003%

Table 1
Summary of results of administration studies with oleander leaves administered in different forms to 2 horses (A and B) and a mule (C)

Animal	Dose (g)	Leaves	Administration Details	Result
A	10	Green	Bran mash	"No perceptible change"
A	25	Green	Capsules	Depression, diarrhea, weakness, inappetence, death in 72 h
B	10	Infusion[a]	Bran mash	Diarrhea within 24 h
B	6	Dry		Diarrhea within 36 h; tachycardia and hyperthermia followed by bradycardia and hypothermia. Critical condition; recovered with "good care."
B	14	Dry		Tachycardia, cold extremities, abdominal pain and sweating, death within 24 h
C	15	Infusion[a]	Full stomach	"Slightly increased pulse"
C	26	Green	Full stomach	Diarrhea, cold extremities, tachycardia, and mild hyperthermia
C	24	Dry	Full stomach	Death within 24 h

Animals: A was a 15 y mare; B was an "old" gelding; and C was an "old" mule.
[a] Infusions were prepared from green leaves macerated and left overnight in distilled water.

body weight) were lethal to adult horses.[14] A gelding administered 6 g dry leaves developed severe clinical signs and was in critical condition but recovered with "good care." A mule administered 26 g green leaves on a full stomach developed diarrhea but recovered. This either could be due to the fact that the mule had recently eaten or could indicate reduced susceptibility of mules compared with horses. Toxic and lethal doses for other cardiac glycoside plants have not been well established in horses.

Clinical Signs, Examination Findings, and Laboratory Confirmation

Common clinical signs of cardiac glycoside poisoning reported in horses, ponies, donkeys, and mules include lethargy, depression, and weakness; inappetence or complete feed refusal; diarrhea; and colic/abdominal pain.[14–16,21–23] Muscle tremors and collapse have also been reported. Mucous membranes can be pale, dark, and/or congested with prolonged capillary refill times. Hyperemic, injected, and toxic mucous membranes have also been reported. Other physical examination findings can include dehydration; weak peripheral pulses and cool extremities; decreased intestinal motility or ileus; decreased anal tone; gaseous distension of the cecum or colon; hyperthermia or hypothermia; and cardiac arrhythmias.[14–16,21–23] Arrhythmias depend on the dose and the time since ingestion and can include bradycardia or tachycardia. Arrhythmias observed on electrocardiography (EKG) include ventricular premature contractions, ventricular tachycardia, third-degree AV block, bundle branch block, and ventricular fibrillation.[15,21–23] In some cases, animals are simply found dead after appearing normal hours prior.

Complications and sequelae of acute toxicosis include acute renal failure; peritoneal, pleural, and/or pericardial effusion; severe colic warranting surgery; pneumonia; and neurologic abnormalities.[21]

Laboratory abnormalities can include elevations in packed cell volume (PCV), total protein, leukocyte count, fibrinogen, blood glucose, creatine kinase (CK), total bilirubin, blood urea nitrogen (BUN), and creatinine. Hyperkalemia may be present early in the disease course.[23]

Postmortem findings in acute cases may be limited to nonspecific lesions associated with heart failure, such as white froth in the nasal passages and tracheal lumen; pulmonary and/or hepatic congestion and edema; hemorrhage and edema of the GI tract, liver, pancreas, adrenal glands, or other organs; and peritoneal, pericardial, and/or pleural effusion.[14–16,] Other lesions can include myocardial necrosis; epicardial, endocardial, or myocardial hemorrhage; enteritis or enterocolitis; hepatocellular necrosis or hepatitis; swollen, pale kidneys; renal tubular necrosis, mineralization, or congestion.[21,24] GI contents, plant material, serum, urine, and feces can be analyzed for cardiac glycosides at some veterinary diagnostic laboratories.[25,26]

Treatment

Gastric lavage via NG tube can be attempted but is unlikely to be rewarding unless performed soon after ingestion. AC seems effective in limiting absorption of cardiac glycosides and may also reduce enterohepatic recirculation and enhance biliary excretion.[4] Cathartics should be used cautiously if at all due to the possibility of exacerbating diarrhea.

Fluid therapy is usually necessary to support cardiovascular function and correct or maintain acid–base and electrolyte balance.[21] Crystalloid fluids should be selected and supplemented based on electrolyte and acid–base status. Colloids and hypertonic saline have also been used in some cases, as has parenteral nutrition.[21]

Antiarrhythmic medications may also be necessary. Phenytoin is considered an "almost specific" antagonist for digitalis-induced ventricular arrhythmias and has been used successfully to convert a Shetland pony with digitalis intoxication[22] and a donkey with oleander intoxication.[23] The pony was treated with a loading dose of 7.5 mg/kg phenytoin IV at 40 mg/min via jugular catheter, which converted ventricular tachycardia into a sinus rhythm.[22] Several hours later ventricular premature beats recurred and oral phenytoin (10 mg/kg) was initiated and continued q 12 hours for 5 days. From days 6 to 14, the dose was adjusted based on the serum digoxin concentration and EKG measurements.[22] The donkey was initially treated with lidocaine, then procainamide, before successful conversion with phenytoin.[23] Although atropine has been used in dogs, it is not recommended in horses due to the risk of severe ileus.

Digoxin-specific Fab antibody fragments (eg, DigiFab, Digibind) have been used successfully in dogs and humans in cases of oleander poisoning.[27] Fab fragments may also be effective in equines; however, cost may limit their use.

Plants

Adonis (pheasant's eye, adonis)
Adonis, or pheasant's eye, species are annual or perennial herbs native to Europe and temperate Asia. Several species have been introduced into North America as ornamentals and are especially popular in rock gardens.[4] *Adonis aestivalis* and *Adonis annua* have escaped cultivation in the western United States and are now abundant in open forests, prairies, and disturbed sites. *Adonis vernalis* occasionally escapes cultivation in the northeastern United States. Plants are erect with solitary red, yellow, or occasionally white flowers, with or without a dark spot in the center and pinnately dissected leaves. Adonis is considered unpalatable, and cases of livestock poisoning are rare; however, horses have been poisoned by contaminated hay.[16,20]

Apocynum cannabinum (dogbane, hemp dogbane)
Dogbanes are perennial herbs distributed throughout North America in dry thickets and forest edges, in ditches, and in open woodlands and fields. Leaves are simple and usually opposite. The small flowers are white, pinkish, or greenish. Mature stems are tough and fibrous, and ingestion of fresh plants is not likely. However, ingestion of tender new shoots could be possible.[4] One reported case occurred in which 2 horses apparently died after ingesting hay contaminated with dogbane.[28]

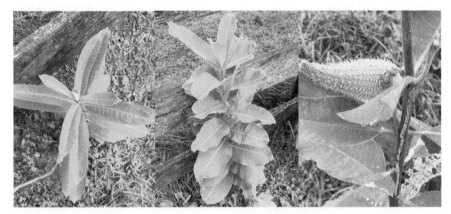

Fig. 2. Common milkweed (*Asclepias syriaca*), a broad-leaved milkweed. Immature leaves (*A*). Mature leaves (*B*). Seedpod, mature leaves with evidence of caterpillar herbivory (*C*).

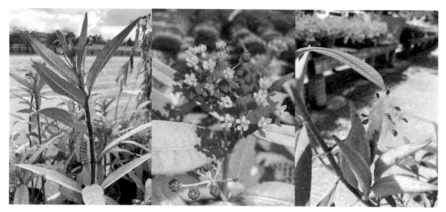

Fig. 3. Bloodflower (*Asclepias curassavica*). Leaves, monarch caterpillar (*A*). Flowers (*B*). Seedpods, seeds with "down" (*C*).

Asclepias (milkweeds)

Milkweeds are herbs with viscous milky white sap from which the common name is derived. Leaves can be broad, narrow, or medium and opposite or whorled (verticillate).[4] Flowers can be solitary or in umbellate clusters, and can be a variety of colors. Various species occur across North America in a wide variety of environments (**Figs. 2–4**). Toxic milkweeds exert either cardiovascular or neurologic effects. Cardiotoxic species include broad-leaved, medium-leaved, and narrow-leaved milkweeds, contrary to the initial division in which broad-leaved plants were considered cardiotoxic and narrow-leaved plants were considered neurotoxic.[4]

All neurotoxic milkweeds identified thus far have been verticillate-leaved, a subset of narrow-leaved milkweeds (**Table 2**). The neurotoxic compound in these plants has not yet been identified.

Cascabela thevetia, previously Thevetia peruviana, Thevetia neriifolia, and Cerbera thevetia (yellow oleander)

Yellow oleander is a shrub or small tree native to the Gulf Coast of Mexico from Tamaulipas through San Luis Potosi but is also found in other tropical regions in the Americas and West Indies.[4] Flower colors range from bright saffron yellow to orange or

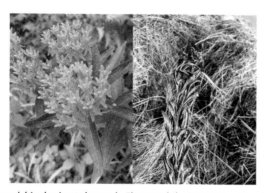

Fig. 4. Butterfly weed (*Asclepias tuberosa*). Flowers (*A*). Contaminating hay (*B*).

Table 2
Neurotoxic verticillate-leaved milkweed (*Asclepias*) species

Scientific Name	Common Name(s)
[a]*A fascicularis*	Narrow-leaved milkweed and Mexican milkweed
[a]*A subverticillata*	Western whorled milkweed and horsetail milkweed
A mexicana	Mexican whorled milkweed
A pumila	Plains whorled milkweed
A verticillata	Eastern whorled milkweed and spider milkweed

[a] Species considered the highest risk.

yellow-pink. Cardenolide concentrations are highest in the seeds and much lower in other plant parts.

Convallaria majalis (lily of the valley)

Lily of the valley, or convallaria, is an herb native to Eurasia and the southern Appalachian Mountains, although populations in North America may represent early naturalizations from European populations.[4] The delicate white, bell-shaped flowers are carried on one-sided raceme (**Fig. 5**). Leaves are basal or subbasal. All parts are toxic, especially the roots.[4] Convallaria is rarely ingested. Poisoning has only occasionally been reported in companion animals and humans; no livestock cases have been reported in the literature.[29]

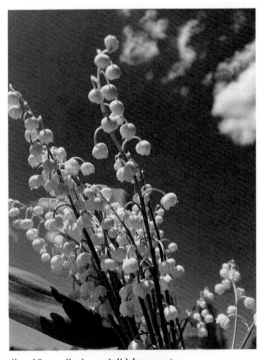

Fig. 5. Lily of the valley (*Convallaria majalis*) bouquet.

Cryptostegia (rubber vine)

Rubber vines are shrubs and woody climbers native to the tropics of Africa, Madagascar, and India, and they are cultivated in frost-free areas of North America. They have escaped cultivation in Florida and have been naturalized in Sinaloa, Mexico.[4] Leaves are oblong elliptical and glossy dark green. The large, funnel-shaped flowers are usually pink or rose-purple but occasionally white. *Cryptostegia* seems palatable, and poisoning has been documented in horses and donkeys.[30] Young leaves seem to be most toxic.

Digitalis (foxglove)

Foxgloves are perennial or biennial herbs native to Europe, northwest Africa, and west central Asia.[4] Several species have been introduced in North America as ornamentals and escaped cultivation. *Digitalis purpurea*, common foxglove, has been widely naturalized in the western third of the continent, particularly the Pacific northwest, as well as the northeast. The characteristic tubular, bell-shaped flowers are carried on elongate racemes.[4] Flowers are pink, purple, bronze, yellow, or white, typically with spots or streaks on the throat.

Cardiac glycosides are present in all parts of the plant, especially the seeds.[4] Concentrations are highest in fruits, flowers, and immature leaves. Livestock are most likely to ingest foxglove in contaminated hay; however, poisoning occurred in ponies turned out into a new field in which *D purpurea* was abundant.[22]

Nerium oleander (oleander, common oleander)

Oleander is a flowering evergreen shrub or small tree with showy, fragrant flowers. Its native range extends from the Mediterranean to western China, although it is now naturalized throughout warmer parts of the world, including the southern United States and Mexico.[4] Its ornamental value and drought tolerance make oleander a popular choice as a hedge, specimen yard plant, and in roadside plantings. Flowers can be white, pink, dark red, or purple (**Fig. 6**A–C). Leaves are leathery and oblong or lanceolate; midrib and secondary veins are prominent.[4] Fresh oleander leaves seem unpalatable; dried leaves and clippings are more palatable, especially when mixed with hay or lawn clippings. Oleander poisoning has been reported in many species, including horses, donkeys, and mules.[14,15,21,23]

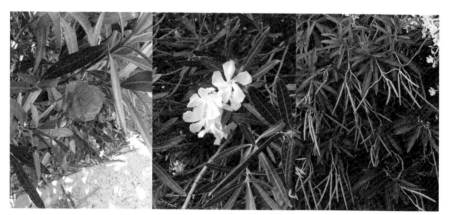

Fig. 6. Oleander (*Nerium oleander*). Pink-flowered, flowers, and leaves (*A*). White-flowered, flowers and leaves (*B*). Leaves and seedpods (*C*).

RHODODENDRONS AND OTHER GRAYANOTOXIN (ERICACEOUS DITERPENOID)-CONTAINING PLANTS

Members of the Ericaceae (heath family) include edible, ornamental, and toxic species. Toxic species contain various ericaceous diterpenoids, often collectively referred to as grayanotoxins.[4] Grayanotoxins are found in all parts of toxic species including the nectar; honey made from such nectar is also toxic. This so-called mad honey is the main problem associated with these plants in humans. Mad honey has caused both accidental and intentional intoxications and has even been used in battle to render enemy troops insensible.[31] Although toxic species are not especially palatable, many are evergreen and may pose a danger in the winter when other food is scarce. Additionally, some species are widely cultivated and therefore abundant in many areas. Although less frequently than sheep, goats, and cattle, horses have occasionally been poisoned by Ericaceae.[32]

Mechanism

Ericaceous diterpenoids bind to sodium channels, especially in excitable cells, slowing channel opening and closing and prolonging activation.[4] Additionally, sodium ion selectivity is decreased, allowing increased permeability to other cations, especially potassium. At very high doses, there may also be effects on calcium channels.

Toxic Dose

Leucothoë are considered the most toxic Ericaceae species, with an estimated toxic dose in sheep as low as 0.12% body weight.[33] Leucothoë are uncommon plants and are less commonly associated with poisoning than the more widely encountered Rhododendron and Kalmia species. Toxic doses are not well established in horses.

Clinical Signs, Examination Findings, and Laboratory Confirmation

Clinical signs of poisoning often develop within several hours of exposure. These can include depression, anorexia, vomiting or regurgitation, hypersalivation and nasal secretions, severe colic/abdominal pain, bloat, and irregular respiration.[32,34–36] Species capable of vomiting can develop persistent retching and vomiting; vomiting may be projectile. Diarrhea is uncommon. Other reported findings include head-pressing, muscle tremors, weakness, recumbency, bradycardia, hypotension, and respiratory depression.[33,34] Acute effects generally resolve within 24 hours if animals survive but weakness and/or neurologic effects can persist for 2 to 3 days.[4] Aspiration pneumonia is a possible sequela, and marked weight loss is possible.

Postmortem examination findings are typically mild and nonspecific.[33] Leaves may be found in the GI tract.[36] Some veterinary diagnostic laboratories can detect grayanotoxins in feces, urine, and GI contents.[37,38]

Treatment

Decontamination and gastric lavage via NG tube can be attempted but is often unrewarding. Administration of AC and a cathartic may help limit toxin absorption. Intravenous lipid emulsion has been used successfully in goats with Pieris intoxication.[36] Supportive care includes intravenous fluid support; analgesia for abdominal pain/colic; and antibiotics if aspiration pneumonia has occurred.

Plants

Representatives of toxic Ericaceae species found in North America are described in this section. Common names and North American ranges are listed in **Table 3**.

Table 3
Representative toxic Ericaceae found in North America

Scientific Name	Common Name	Range in North America
Andromeda		
A polifolia (A glaucophylla)	Bog rosemary, marsh Andromeda, and andromeda	Sphagnum peat bogs and wet, acidic sites in Canada and the northeastern United States
Eubotrys		
E racemosa	Fetterbush, swamp fetterbush, calfkill, kill-calf, deciduous, and swamp doghobble	Eastern United States, moist acidic soils of woods and barrens of eastern coastal plains
E recurva	Deciduous mountain fetterbush, and redtwig doghobble	Eastern United States, moist woods at higher elevations
Kalmia		
K angustifolia	Sheep laurel, lambkill, wicky, sheep poison, lamb laurel, low laurel, and dwarf laurel	Newfoundland to Georgia along the edges of bogs and swamps and in moist, acidic soils of coastal plains and mountains
K latifolia	Mountain laurel, laurel, calico bush, ivybush, spoonwood, sheep laurel, poison laurel, small laurel, rose laurel, high laurel, and roundleaf laurel	Maine to Florida; most abundant in Appalachian Mountains. Dense thickets in sandy, rocky, acidic soils of lowland hills, stream banks, slopes, and mountainsides
K microphylla	Small-leaved laurel, alpine laurel, bog laurel, western swamp laurel, western swamp kalmia, pale laurel, and western laurel	Subalpine and alpine mountain meadows primarily in western North America
K polifolia	Swamp laurel and bog laurel	Bogs and moist meadows from Alaska to Labrador
Leucothoë		
L axillaris	Dog laurel, hemlock, calfkill, leucothoe, swamp dog laurel, and coastal doghobble	Eastern and western United States
L davisiae	Black laurel and sierra laurel	Western North America, wet areas with acidic soils in the Sierra Nevada and Cascade Mountains
L fontanesiana	Drooping leucothoe, mountain dog-laurel, and highland doghobble	Mountain streams
Lyonia		
L ligustrina	Maleberry, male blueberry, he-huckleberry, and big-boy	Eastern United States to Texas and Oklahoma, swamps and wet areas
L mariana	Staggerbush and Piedmont staggerbush	Eastern United States, moist sandy sites

(continued on next page)

Table 3
(continued)

Scientific Name	Common Name	Range in North America
Menziesia		
M ferruginea	Rusty menziesia, rusty-leaved menziesia, mock azalea, fool's huckleberry, tree lyonia, smooth pacific menziesia, and false azalea	Woods and stream banks especially north slopes of hillsides. Rocky and Sierra-Cascade Mountains
M pilosa	Minniebush	Appalachian Mountains
Pieris		
P floribunda	Fetterbush, mountain fetterbush, and mountainpieris	Mountain woods of eastern United States
P japonica	Lily-of-the-valley bush and Japanese pieris	Eastern North America, cultivated as an ornamental
Rhododendron		
R albiflorum	White rhododendron and cascade rhododendron	Western half of North America
R catawbiense	Mountain rosebay, red laurel, purple laurel, rosebay laurel, and Catawba rhododendron	Eastern quarter of North America
R columbianum	Western Labrador tea, trapper's tea, and smooth Labrador tea	Western half of North America
R groenlandicum	Bog Labrador tea, common Labrador tea	Northern third of North America
R macrophyllum	Pacific rhododendron, western rhododendron, and California rosebay	Western half of North America
R maximum	Rosebay, great laurel, and white laurel	Eastern quarter of North America
R occidentale	Western azalea	Western half of North America
R tomentosum	Northern Labrador tea, marsh Labrador tea	Northern third of North America

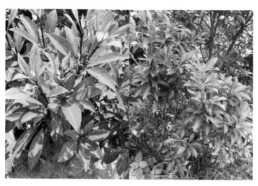

Fig. 7. Mountain laurel (*Kalmia latifolia*). Immature (*A*). Mature (*B*).

Andromeda polifolia
Evergreen shrubs with white or pink urn-shaped flowers.[4]

Eubotrys species
Deciduous shrubs or small trees with white tubular, ovoid, or urn-shaped or bell-shaped flowers.[4]

Kalmia species
Evergreen or deciduous shrubs or small trees (**Fig. 7**A and B). Flowers can be bell-shaped or round and have white, pink, light rose, or rose purple petals with a red ring at the base of the lobes.[4]

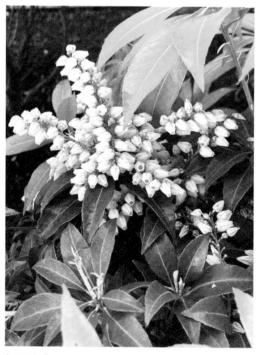

Fig. 8. Pieris (*Pieris japonica*).

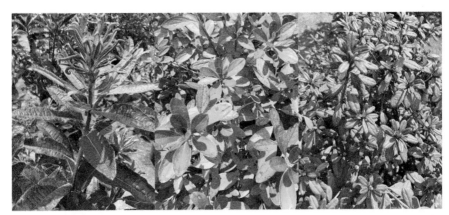

Fig. 9. Various *Rhododendron x* (*Azalea*) cultivars. "Klondyke" azalea (*A*). "Karen" azalea (*B*). White azalea (*C*).

Leucothoë species
Evergreen shrubs or small trees with white tubular, ovoid, or urn-shaped or bell-shaped flowers.[4] Similar in appearance to the deciduous *Eubotrys*.

Lyonia species
Evergreen or deciduous shrubs or rarely small trees with cylindrical or urn-shaped or bell-shaped flowers.[4] Petals are white, pink, or rose.

Pieris species
Evergreen shrubs or small trees with fragrant white or pink flowers.[4] Flowers are carried on panicles or racemes, often 1-sided (**Fig. 8**).

Rhododendron species
Shrubs or rarely small trees widely cultivated as ornamentals. Most evergreen species are known as rhododendrons, and most deciduous species are known as azaleas.[4] Other common names for *Rhododendron* species include rosebays, laurels, and Labrador teas. Flowers can be round, bell-shaped, or funnel-shaped and can be most colors except blue (**Fig. 9**A–C).[4]

CLINICS CARE POINTS

- Some toxic landscaping plants are unpalatable fresh but readily accepted dried, especially when mixed into hay or lawn clippings
- Horses are most often exposed when plant trimmings or clippings are discarded within reach or fed intentionally by well-meaning owners or neighbors
- Some plants may cause only GI upset; others can be fatal even in small amounts
- Treatment can be unrewarding due to the acute, rapidly progressive nature of poisoning, so client education aimed at prevention is critical
- AC with or without cathartics may be useful in recent ingestions
- Digoxin Fab fragments have been used successfully in oleander toxicosis in a dog but may be prohibitively expensive in horses
- No antidote is available for most toxic plant ingestions, and treatment is symptomatic and supportive

DISCLOSURE

The author has nothing to disclose.

REFERENCES

1. Gurib-Fakim A. Medicinal plants: traditions of yesterday and drugs of tomorrow. Mol Aspects Med 2006;27(1):1–93.
2. Alden CL, Fosnaugh CJ, Smith JB, et al. Japanese yew poisoning of large domestic animals in the Midwest. J Am Vet Med Assoc 1977;170(3):314–6.
3. Parkinson N. Yew poisoning in horses. Can Vet J 1996;37(11):687. https://www.ncbi.nlm.nih.gov/pmc/articles/PMC1576505/pdf/canvetj00108-0049.pdf.
4. Burrows GE, Tyrl RJ. Toxic plants of north America. 2nd edition. Ames, IA: John Wiley & Sons; 2013.
5. Wilson CR, Sauer JM, Hooser SB. Taxines: a review of the mechanism and toxicity of yew (*Taxus* spp.) alkaloids. Toxicon 2001;39(2–3):175–85.
6. Lowe JE, Hintz HF, Schryver HF, Kingsbury JM. Taxus cuspidata (Japanese yew) poisoning in horses. Cornell Vet. 1970;60:36–39. Cited by: Veatch JK, Reid FM, Kennedy GA. Differentiating yew poisoning from other toxicoses. Veterinary medicine (USA). 1988;298–239.
7. Todorov T, Stamberov P, Nikolov B, et al. Fatal European yew (*Taxus baccata*) poisoning in two horses. Tradition and Modernity in Veterinary Medicine 2019; 4(2):7. http://scij-tmvm.com/vol./vol.4/2/vol-4-2_2019-34-39.pdf.
8. Cope RB, Camp C, Lohr CV. Fatal yew (*Taxus* sp) poisoning in Willamette Valley, Oregon, horses. Vet Hum Toxicol 2004;46(5):279–81.
9. Tiwary AK, Puschner B, Kinde H, et al. Diagnosis of Taxus (yew) poisoning in a horse. J Vet Diagn Invest 2005;17(3):252–5. https://journals.sagepub.com/doi/pdf/10.1177/104063870501700307.
10. Froldi R, Croci PF, Dell'Acqua L, et al. Preliminary gas chromatography with mass spectrometry determination of 3, 5-dimethoxyphenol in biological specimens as evidence of taxus poisoning. J Anal Toxicol 2010;34(1):53–6.
11. Burcham GN, Becker KJ, Tahara JM, et al. Myocardial fibrosis associated with previous ingestion of yew (*Taxus* sp.) in a Holstein heifer: evidence for chronic yew toxicity in cattle. J Vet Diagn Invest 2013;25(1):147–52.
12. Burchell HB. Digitalis poisoning: historical and forensic aspects. J Am Coll Cardiol 1983;1(2):506–16.
13. Patel S. Plant-derived cardiac glycosides: role in heart ailments and cancer management. Biomed Pharmacother 2016;84:1036–41.
14. Wilson FW. Oleander poisoning of live-stock. University of Arizona Agricultural Experiment Station bulletin 59. 1909. Available at: https://play.google.com/books/reader?id=V8oe_KzgwKkC&pg=GBS.PA382. Accessed August 31, 2023.
15. Hughes KJ, Dart AJ, Hodgson DR. Suspected *Nerium oleander* (Oleander) poisoning in a horse. Aust Vet J 2002;80(7):412–5.
16. Woods LW, Filigenzi MS, Booth MC, et al. Summer pheasant's eye (*Adonis aestivalis*) poisoning in three horses. Vet Pathol 2004;41(3):215–20.
17. Jortani SA, Helm RA, Valdes R Jr. Inhibition of Na, K-ATPase by oleandrin and oleandrigenin, and their detection by digoxin immunoassays. Clin Chem 1996; 42(10):1654–8.
18. Rose AM, Valdes R Jr. Understanding the sodium pump and its relevance to disease. Clin Chem 1994;40(9):1674–85.

19. Suhail M. Na, K-ATPase: ubiquitous multifunctional transmembrane protein and its relevance to various pathophysiological conditions. J Clin Med Res 2010; 2(1):1–17.
20. Degen AV, Adonis-vergiftung. Fortschr Landwirtsch. 1932;7:556. Cited by: Woods LW, Filigenzi MS, Booth MC, et al. Summer pheasant's eye (Adonis aestivalis) poisoning in three horses. Vet Pathol. 2004;41(3):215–220.
21. Renier AC, Kass PH, Magdesian KG, et al. Oleander toxicosis in equids: 30 cases (1995–2010). J Am Vet Med Assoc 2013;242(4):540–9.
22. Wijnberg D, Van Der Kolk JH, Hiddink EG. Use of phenytoin to treat digitalis-induced cardiac arrhythmias in a miniature Shetland pony. Vet Rec 1999; 144(10):259–61.
23. Smith PA, Aldridge BM, Kittleson MD. Oleander toxicosis in a donkey. J Vet Intern Med 2003;17(1):111–4. Available at: https://www.researchgate.net/profile/Mark-Kittleson/publication/10919273_Oleander_Toxicosis_in_a_Donkey/links/5af1c44ba ca272bf42562be2/Oleander-Toxicosis-in-a-Donkey.pdf.
24. Sykes CA, Uzal FA, Mete A, et al. Renal lesions in horses with oleander (*Nerium oleander*) poisoning. Animals 2022;12(11):1443.
25. Galey FD, Holstege DM, Plumlee KH, et al. Diagnosis of oleander poisoning in livestock. J Vet Diagn Invest 1996;8(3):358–64.
26. Filigenzi MS, Woods LW, Booth MC, et al. Determination of strophanthidin in ingesta and plant material by LC-MS/MS. J Agric Food Chem 2004;52(8):2174–8.
27. Pao-Franco A, Hammond TN, Weatherton LK, et al. Successful use of digoxin-specific immune Fab in the treatment of severe *Nerium oleander* toxicosis in a dog. J Vet Emerg Crit Care 2017;27(5):596–604.
28. Fuller TC, McClintock EM. Poisonous plants of California. Univ of California Press; 1986. Cited by Burrows G.E. and Tyrl R.J., Toxic plants of north America 2nd edition, 2013, John Wiley & Sons; Ames, IA
29. Berny P, Caloni F, Croubels S, et al. Animal poisoning in Europe. Part 2: companion animals. Vet J 2010;183(3):255–9.
30. Cook DR, Campbell GW, Meldrum AR. Suspected *Cryptostegia grandiflora* (rubber vine) poisoning in horses. Aust Vet J 1990;67(9):344.
31. Jansen SA, Kleerekooper I, Hofman ZL, et al. Grayanotoxin poisoning: 'mad honey disease' and beyond. Cardiovasc Toxicol 2012;12:208–15.
32. Knight AP, Walter RG. A guide to plant poisoning of animals in North America. Jackson, WY: Teton New Media; 2002.
33. Crawford AC, Mountain L. A poisonous plant. US Department of agriculture bureau of plant industry bulletin 121, part 2. Washington: US Government Printing Office; 1908. Available at: https://play.google.com/books/reader?id=9soaAA AAYAAJ&pg=GBS.PA13&hl=en. Accessed 9 April, 2023.
34. Puschner B, Holstege DM, Lamberski N. Grayanotoxin poisoning in three goats. J Am Vet Med Assoc 2001;218(4):573–5.
35. Pischon H, Petrick A, Müller M, et al. Grayanotoxin I intoxication in pet pigs. Vet Pathol 2018;55(6):896–9.
36. Bischoff K, Smith MC, Stump S. Treatment of pieris ingestion in goats with intravenous lipid emulsion. J Med Toxicol 2014;10:411–4.
37. Holstege DM, Francis T, Puschner B, et al. Multiresidue screen for cardiotoxins by two-dimensional thin-layer chromatography. J Agric Food Chem 2000;48(1):60–4.
38. Holstege DM, Puschner B, Le T. Determination of grayanotoxins in biological samples by LC-MS/MS. J Agric Food Chem 2001;49(3):1648–51.

Pyrogallol Toxicosis in Horses

Karyn Bischoff, DVM, MS, MPH

KEYWORDS

- Red maple • *Acer rubrum* • Pyrogallol • *Pistacia* spp • Anemia • Heinz body
- Methemoglobinemia

KEY POINTS

- Acute hemolysis has been reported in horses that ingest wilted maple (*Acer* spp) leaves, and particularly red maple leaves (*Acer rubrum*) in the summer or autumn, and in horses that ingest *Pistacia* spp leaves or seeds.
- Pyrogallol, produced by metabolism of gallic acid from *Acer* spp leaves and *Pistacia* spp seeds by equine enteric microflora, is thought to be the causative agent of hemolysis and methemoglobinemia in horses.
- Symptomatic and supportive care, including early gastrointestinal decontamination, fluid therapy, oxygen supplementation, and pain control, are the mainstays of therapy.
- The prognosis is guarded to poor, and fewer than half of affected horses are expected to survive.

INTRODUCTION

Red maple (*Acer rubrum*; **Fig. 1**) has been implicated most frequently in acute methemoglobinemia and hemolytic crisis in horses, although suspect cases in other species were associated with hybrid species.[1] There are 13 *Acer* species in North America, including box elders, sugar maple, and silver maple, and they are found across the eastern half of the United States.[2] Leaves and especially seeds from the pistachio trees, *Pistacia atlantica*, *Pistacia terebinthus*, and *Pistacia chinensis*, have been observed to cause a similar clinical syndrome in horses.[3,4] Pistachio trees are cultivated in warm, arid areas of the United States.[2,4]

HISTORY

Acute hemolytic anemia due to red maple ingestion was first discovered on horse farms in the United States in New York, Pennsylvania, and areas of New England.[5]

Department of Population Medicine and Diagnostic Sciences, Cornell University College of Veterinary Medicine, New York State Animal Health Diagnostic Center, PO Box 5786, Ithaca, NY 14853, USA
E-mail address: KLB72@cornell.edu

Vet Clin Equine 40 (2024) 77–82
https://doi.org/10.1016/j.cveq.2023.10.001
0749-0739/24/© 2023 Elsevier Inc. All rights reserved.

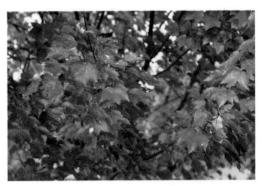

Fig. 1. Canopy of *A rubrum*, red maple trees. (Courtesy of Karan Agrawal).

Similar cases were soon reported in Georgia and New Jersey.[6,7] Eventually, more cases were reported throughout the North American range of red maple, as well as in the southwestern part of the United States where pistachio trees are found.[3,8] Red maple hybrids and, potentially, other species of maple (*Acer* spp) may also induce hemolytic anemia.[8,9] Anemic horses with red maple toxicosis were seen between June and October and had Heinz body formation, methemoglobinemia, or both.[5] Affected horses in early reports seemed malnourished and were consuming poor quality feed.[7] There was no predilection for maple toxicosis based on age, breed, or sex. Confirmation of red maple as the culprit occurred when leaves and bark from red maple trees on affected farms were collected and fed to 2 ponies, which both became affected by hemolysis within 48 hours and were dead within 6 days.[5] Since then, red maple has been implicated in hemolytic disease in Grevy's zebra, another equid, and in alpacas.[1,8]

DISCUSSION
Toxicity

- Fresh red maple leaves fed to ponies did not result in clinical signs.[7]
- Dried red maple leaves were toxic to ponies at a dose of 1.5 g/kg body weight.[6,7]
- Freezing did not alter toxicity and dried leaves remained toxic for at least 30 days.[7]
- Leaves collected after September 15 were lethal within 18 hours, whereas leaves collected earlier in the summer caused death after 2 to 5 days of clinical toxicosis.[7]

Hydrolysable tannins in red maple were considered the likely cause of oxidative damage to erythrocytes.[2] Further evidence has determined that gallic acid is metabolized by microbes identified as *Klebsiella pneumoniae* and *Enterobacter cloacae*, both of which are found in the environment and in the equine ileum, to pyrogallol (**Fig. 2**), potentially through an intermediate compound.[9] Pyrogallol is a potent oxidant, and a concentration of 25 μg/mL in equine blood caused visually apparent methemoglobin formation.[9]

Oxidative stress causes oxidation of hemoglobin to methemoglobin, which decreases oxygen carrying capacity, and Heinz body formation, which increases erythrocyte fragility, leading to hemolysis.[7] Horses have a limited methemoglobin reductase activity.[7] Mechanisms exist for reducing methemoglobin: glutathione is an important scavenger of reactive oxygen species, and methemoglobin reductase, a nicotinamide adenine dinucleotide phosphate-dependent enzyme, reduces methemoglobin; however, these mechanisms for detoxification become rapidly depleted in horses exposed

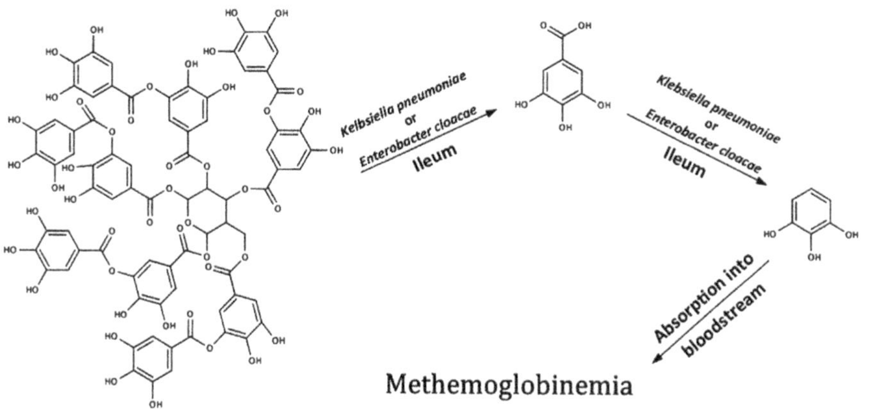

Methemoglobinemia

Fig. 2. Proposed pathway of red maple toxicosis. (Courtesy of Karan Agrawal).

to red maple leaves.[7,10,11] Horses have both reduced activity of methemoglobin reductase compared to other livestock and reduced ability to regenerate glutathione.[4] Peracute death in horses has been associated with rapid onset of tissue hypoxia due to methemoglobinemia in red maple poisoning.[10] Decreased hematocrit also leads to tissue hypoxia, and intravascular hemolysis can cause hemoglobinuric nephrosis in horses that survive the initial insult.[7]

Clinical signs

Clinical signs reported in horses exposed to wilted red maple or pistachio leaves are mostly attributable to hemolytic crisis.[7] Horses that died within 18 hours of red maple ingestion were clinically obtunded and cyanosis was observed.[7] Equids that survived longer became obtunded, refused feed, and presented with cyanosis, brown urine, and icterus on the first day.[7,10] Pregnant mares have aborted.[11]

- Hematocrit and erythrocyte count decreased after the first day postexposure, Heinz bodies and spherocytes became detectable, and methemoglobin concentration increased in the blood.[7,10]
- Fever was intermittent.[10]
- Urine on day 2 contained hemoglobin, methemoglobin, protein, and bilirubin.[7]
- Clinical signs progressed the next day to include icterus, brown blood (due to methemoglobinemia), and increased respiratory and heart rates.[7]
- Heinz body numbers increased until day 3.[7]
- White blood cell counts increased by day 3, as did plasma concentrations of unconjugated and total bilirubin, creatinine, urea nitrogen, aspartate aminotransferase, sorbitol dehydrogenase, and total protein.[1,7]
- Most deaths occurred within 6 days postexposure, when cyanosis and hemoglobinuria had resolved.[7]

A study of 32 affected horses[12] found the following:

- Anemia present in 97% of those with hematocrit taken at initial examination (29/30),
- Renal insufficiency in 41% and colic in 43%,
- Heinz bodies were seen in 33% of initial bloodwork samples,
- Laminitis was reported in 32% of horses with red maple toxicosis.[12]

Postmortem Lesions

- Peracute deaths were associated with a brown cast to the tissues on postmortem examination, suggesting methemoglobinemia.[7]
- Pulmonary edema and hepatic lipidosis were seen histologically, and hemorrhage was noted in the adrenal cortex.[7]
- Equids that died after 3 days had icterus, serosal petechia and ecchymosis, enlarged spleens, and nutmeg liver.[7]
- Microscopic changes included erythrophagia in splenic macrophages and hemoglobinuric nephrosis.[7,8]
- Centrilobular hepatic necrosis was reported in an affected zebra.[8]
- A study that included postmortem examination of 6 horses found the following:
  - 6 out of 6 had icterus,
  - 4 out of 6 had splenomegaly,
  - 3 out of 6 had serosal petechia,
  - 2 out of 6 had affected ceca,
  - 2 out of 6 had pigmentary nephrosis,
  - 1 out of 6 had pulmonary edema,
  - 1 out of 6 had typhlocolitis.[12]

Diagnosis

Diagnosis of red maple or pistachio tree toxicosis in equids is usually based on exposure to the plant in the late summer and early fall, especially fallen branches with wilted leaves, and appropriate clinical signs, clinical pathology, anatomic pathology changes, and ruling out other causes. Wilted maple leaves in the spring were associated with toxicosis in alpacas.[1]

Laboratory testing can be used to support the diagnosis. Spectrophotometric assay has been used to determine circulating methemoglobin concentrations in affected animals.[8] Pyrogallol has been detected in the urine of horses ingesting pistachios.[3,4]

Differential diagnoses can include equine infectious anemia, immune-mediated hemolytic anemia, ingestion of Allium spp (onions, garlic, and chives), piroplasmosis, leptospirosis, ehrlichiosis, phenothiazine toxicosis, and congenital methemoglobinemia.[10,11]

Treatment

Early diagnosis and treatment are critical to survival in affected animals.[1,10]

- Gastric lavage soon after ingestion, instillation of activated charcoal by nasogastric tube, and both have been attempted to prevent toxin absorption.[1,10]
  - Activated charcoal can be given at a dose of 1 to 3 g/kg body weight.
- Supportive care is the mainstay of treatment of equids and other species with red maple or pistachio tree toxicosis.
  - Fluids are given to correct dehydration and electrolyte imbalances and to improve renal perfusion.[10,11]
  - Oxygen may be provided to improve tissue oxygenation.[10]
  - Transfusions have been used to treat severe anemia (hematocrit <12%).[8,10] Whole blood transfusion was not associated with an increased likelihood of survival but this may be because transfused patients were already severely compromised.[12]
  - Sedation may be needed for fractious patients.[10]
  - Nonsteroidal anti-inflammatory drugs (NSAIDS) can be used for pain control and to treat or prevent fever.[10] Pain control is critical because many horses present with signs of colic and inflammation.[12]

Methylene blue is frequently used to treat methemoglobinemia in other species but has not proved to be useful in red maple toxicosis in horses.[10] Vitamin C (ascorbic acid) has also been used to treat methemoglobinemia in horses exposed to red maple either at a dose of 125 mg/kg PO and 40 mg/kg subcutaneously twice daily or intravascularly at 30 to 50 mg/kg IV twice per day but did not increase the likelihood of survival.[10,12] The use of corticosteroids significantly decreased the likelihood of survival.[10,12]

The prognosis for horses with red maple toxicosis is guarded; between 59% and 65% of horses will not survive.[1] A study determined that pyrexia was associated with survival in horses that were poisoned by red maple but this may be because pyrexia occurs relatively late in the progression of clinical signs, beyond the timeline for mortality.[12]

Because of the poor prognosis, the need for aggressive therapy, and the impacts on animal welfare, preventing horses from accessing maple or pistachio trees is the best protective measure.

SUMMARY

It was discovered that red maple was toxic to horses in the early 1980s.[6,7] Since that time, other plants in the maple genus, *Acer*, as well as plants in the pistachio genus, *Pistacia*, have been reported to cause similar clinical signs and lesions in horses.[3,4] Furthermore, toxicosis has been reported in other equids and in camelids.[1,8] The cause of red maple toxicosis is complex and seems to be the metabolism of gallic acids from maple leaves to pyrogallol by enteric bacteria of the horse.[9] Pyrogallol is a potent oxidant that acts on hemoglobin to produce methemoglobin and Heinz bodies, leading to the clinical presentation of cyanosis, anemia, and hemoglobinuria.[9,12] Diagnosis is often tentative and circumstantial, based on evidence of exposure and appropriate clinical signs, although pyrogallol has been detected in urine of clinically affected horses.[3]

Treatment of red maple toxicosis is symptomatic and supportive and can include detoxification with activated charcoal per nasogastric tube; fluid therapy to maintain blood volume, correct electrolyte abnormalities, and provide renal support; supplemental oxygen; and NSAIDS for pain control.[10,11] The use of corticosteroids and antioxidants such as vitamin C and methylene blue do not improve prognosis.[10,12] Prognosis is guarded to poor but horses that survive 6 days postexposure are expected to recover.[1,7,12]

CLINICS CARE POINTS

- Detoxification
  - Gastric lavage for recent ingestion or instillation of activated charcoal may decrease absorption.
- Supportive care
  - Fluid therapy to prevent dehydration, correct electrolyte abnormalities, and prevent hemoglobinuric nephrosis.
  - Oxygen supplementation.
  - Transfusion may be necessary for severe anemia but circulating pyrogallol can potentially hemolyze supplemental erythrocytes.
  - Antioxidants have not proven helpful.
  - NSAIDS are usually needed for pain control.
  - Corticosteroids are contraindicated.

82Bischoff

- Prognosis
  - Only about a third of cases survive.
  - Horses that develop elevated body temperatures are more likely to survive.
  - Horses alive 6 days postexposure are likely to survive.

DISCLOSURE

The author has nothing to disclose.

REFERENCES

1. Dewitt SF, Bedenice D, Mazan MR. Hemolysis and Heinz body formation associated with ingestion of red maple leaves in two alpacas. J Am Vet Med Assoc 2004;225:578–83, 539.
2. Burrows GE, Tyrl RJ. Toxic Plants of North America. 2nd edition. Ames, Iowa: John Wiley & Sons, Inc.; 2013.
3. Bozorgmanesh R, Magdesian KG, Rhodes DM, et al. Hemolytic anemia in horses associated with ingestion of Pistacia leaves. J Vet Intern Med 2015;29:410–3.
4. Walter KM, Moore CE, Bozorgmanesh R, et al. Oxidant-induced damage to equine erythrocytes from exposure to *Pistacia atlantica, Pistacia terebinthus,* and *Pistacia chinensis.* J Vet Diagn Invest 2014;26:821–6.
5. Tennant B, Dill SG, Glickman LT, et al. Acute hemolytic anemia, methemoglobinemia, and Heinz body formation associated with ingestion of red maple leaves by horses. J Am Vet Med Assoc 1981;179:143–50.
6. Divers TJ, George LW, George JW. Hemolytic anemia in horses after the ingestion of red maple leaves. J Am Vet Med Assoc 1982;180:300–2.
7. George LW, Divers TJ, Mahaffey EA, et al. Heinz body anemia and methemoglobinemia in ponies given red maple (*Acer rubrum* L.) leaves. Vet Pathol 1982;19:521–33.
8. Weber M, Miller RE. Presumptive red maple (*Acer rubrum*) toxicosis in Grevy's zebra (Equus grevyi). J Zoo Wildl Med 1997;28:105–8.
9. Agrawal K, Ebel JG, Altier C, et al. Identification of protoxins and a microbial basis for red maple (*Acer rubrum*) toxicosis in equines. J Vet Diagn Invest 2013;25:112–9.
10. McConnico RS, Brownie CF. The use of ascorbic acid in the treatment of 2 cases of red maple (*Acer rubrum*)-poisoned horses. Cornell Vet 1992;82:293–300.
11. Stair EL, Edwards WC, Burrows GE, et al. Suspected red maple (*Acer rubrum*) toxicosis with abortion in two Percheron mares. Vet Hum Toxicol 1993;35:229–30.
12. Alward A, Corriher CA, Barton MH, et al. Red maple (*Acer rubrum*) leaf toxicosis in horses: a retrospective study of 32 cases. J Vet Intern Med 2006;20:1197–201.

Other biotoxins (mycotoxins, cantharidin, cyanobacteria, and snake envenomations)

Equine Mycotoxins

Steve Ensley, DVM, PhD[a], Michelle Mostrom, DVM, MS, PhD[b],*

KEYWORDS

- Mycotoxins • Aflatoxin • Fumonisins • Trichothecenes • Deoxynivalenol • T-2 toxin
- Zearalenone • Equine

KEY POINTS

- Feed refusal by equine is often the first clinical sign observed by owners and should immediately trigger removal of feed and further inspection of the ration, with possible analysis for toxins by a veterinary diagnostic laboratory.
- Few mycotoxins have an antidote, and treatment involves removal of the contaminated feed and replacement with a "clean" feed with supportive care for the clinical signs.
- Feeding corn dried distillers' grains to equine is contra-indicated due to the concentration of fumonisins (and possibly aflatoxins) in the by-product and because equine are very sensitive to fumonisins causing adverse effects. Do not feed corn screenings to equine, and in drought years analyze corn and corn products for fumonisins.

INTRODUCTION

Mold growth and subsequent production of secondary metabolites or mycotoxins can occur in cereal grains, pasture grasses, hays, and straws under specific conditions of moisture and temperature. Some of these mycotoxins primarily occur in the field and others can develop under storage conditions. Mold growth and mycotoxin production are typically greater in drought stressed or damaged crops and (1) feeding these poorer quality products, (2) often feeding cereal byproducts that can concentrate mycotoxins, or (3) feeding corn screenings increases the risk of mycotoxicosis in equine. The main mycotoxins involved in adverse equine health issues are aflatoxins, trichothecenes, fumonisins, zearalenone and the endophyte-produced ergovaline in fescue grass. This article is focused on the more common mycotoxins occurring in feeds provided to equine.

[a] Veterinary Diagnostic Laboratory, College of Veterinary Medicine, Kansas State University, P217 Mosier Hall, 1800 Denison Avenue, Manhattan, KS 66506, USA; [b] North Dakota State University, Veterinary Diagnostic Laboratory, 4035 19th Avenue North, Department 7691 P.O. Box 6050, Fargo, North Dakota 58108-6050, USA
* Corresponding author.
E-mail address: michelle.mostrom@ndsu.edu

Vet Clin Equine 40 (2024) 83–94
https://doi.org/10.1016/j.cveq.2023.10.002
0749-0739/24/© 2023 Elsevier Inc. All rights reserved.

Aflatoxins

Aflatoxin contamination of horse feed is probably underreported.[1] There is not much information in the literature about clinical aflatoxicosis in horses. Liver damage in horses should always include aflatoxin in the differential list.

The Food and Drug Administration (FDA) legally regulates the concentration of aflatoxin allowed in feed for human and animal consumption because it is a known carcinogen. Aflatoxin B_1 (AFB_1) causes mutagenicity by forming AFB_1 8,9-epoxide. Several forms of cytochrome (CYP) P450 such as CYP 3A4 and 2A6 will catalyze the activation of AFB_1 to AFB_1 8,9-epoxide. This epoxide reacts with DNA to form persistent adducts. AFB_1 also inhibits protein synthesis interfering with the formation of enzymes necessary for energy, metabolism, and fat mobilization. The different toxicosis seen in different species is caused by the species differences in activation and detoxification processes of the metabolite, AFB_1 reactive epoxide. The formation of DNA-bound AFB_1 metabolites by liver microsomes has been demonstrated, leading to AFB_1 in the horse liver.

FDA publishes a legal action level for aflatoxins in animal feed in a compliance policy guide. The guidelines are in Section 683.100.[2] The guidelines for horses are under the intended use category of "Dairy animals and other animal species." The food ingredient category includes corn, peanut products, cottonseed meal, and other animal food and food ingredients with an aflatoxin action level (maximum inclusion) of 20 ppb (part per billion or $\mu g/kg$). Aflatoxin has been found in many feeds in different countries. Gunsen and Yaroglu collected 20 samples of equine feed in Turkey.[3] Two/twenty feed samples in this study exceeded the Turkish tolerance of aflatoxin of 10 ppb. Keller and colleagues collected equine feed samples in Brazil from June 2003 to March 2004.[4] Elevated concentrations of aflatoxin and fumonisin were detected in these feeds as well.

The target organ for aflatoxin in all species is the liver. *Aspergillus flavus* and *Aspergillus parasiticus* produce aflatoxins in human and animal food. Other less common molds include *A niger, A wentii, Penicillium citrinum,* and *P frequentans*. Aflatoxins are composed of B1, B2, G1, and G2. AFB_1 is the most common, most potent, and the one we have the most information about. AFB_1 is the most potent hepatocarcinogen of the four aflatoxins. The abbreviations B and G for aflatoxin come from the color of the mold's fluorescence under ultraviolet light. The aflatoxin molds are blue and green.

Aflatoxin M1 is a metabolite of aflatoxin and can be detected in milk and tissues. Clinical signs of aflatoxicosis include reduced appetite, depression, increased body temperature, tremors, ataxia, and other nonspecific clinical signs. Necropsy findings can include a yellow to brown liver with centrilobular necrosis, icterus, hemorrhage, and brown urine.

The production of aflatoxins in feeds is directly related to drought. As the climate gets hotter and dryer, more aflatoxin will be produced in the grains we use for horse feed. The optimum temperature for growth for *Aspergillus* is 25°C to 30°C (77°–86° F) with a relative humidity of 97% to 99%. All the grains and grain products we feed horses have the potential to be contaminated with aflatoxin. Aflatoxin is a class 1B carcinogen, the most potent hepatocarcinogen known. It can cause acute and chronic toxicosis, carcinogenicity, teratogenicity, genotoxicity, and immunotoxicity.

A total dietary concentration of 500 to 1000 $\mu g/kg$ (ppb) has been shown to cause adverse health in horses.[5] In another study in ponies, adverse health was noted at 0.3 mg/kg or ppm (part per million that converts to 300 $\mu g/kg$ or ppb) aflatoxin in feed.

In addition to liver, other tissues may be affected by aflatoxin exposure. A possible link between aflatoxicosis and chronic obstructive pulmonary disease (COPD) was found by Larsson and colleagues.[6] COPD was also associated with inhaled mycotoxins.[7] *A fumigatus* and *Micropolyspora faeni* are potential causes of COPD in horses. The inhaled aflatoxins and other xenobiotics may be activated by CYP enzymes in the epithelial linings of the respiratory tract and contribute to the etiology of COPD.[5]

There is no specific treatment or antidote for aflatoxin. Treatment is based on clinical signs.

Fumonisins

Equine leukoencephalomalacia (ELEM) was reported from consumption of contaminated corn in 1902,[8] from cultures of *Fusarium moniliforme* in 1971,[9] and with a study of a pure compound of Fumonisin B1 in 1988.[10] Fumonisins are produced by *Fusarium verticillioides*, *Fusarium proliferatum,* and other *Fusarium* species.[11] Fumonisins are commonly found in corn and corn byproducts. ELEM has been called moldy corn poisoning, blind staggers, corn stalk disease, and circling disease. Dried distillers' grain with solubles is a common ingredient in animal feeds that often contains elevated concentrations of fumonisins. Corn screening can contain high fumonisin concentrations and should not be fed to horses unless tested for fumonisins.

Horses are the most sensitive species to fumonisin. The FDA guidelines for fumonisin in horse feeds are for fumonisin B1[FB1]+FB2+FB3 to have a total of 5 ppm in no more than 20% of the diet on a dry matter basis.[12] This is effectively no more than 1 ppm in the diet of a horse. *Fusarium* is a field toxin rather than a storage mycotoxin. FB1 is toxic to the liver in all species and the kidney in a range of laboratory and farm animals. FB1 can also damage the heart of horses. Fumonisins inhibit ceramide synthase in all species and disrupt sphingolipid metabolism. This causes a disruption of endothelial cell membranes. In swine, fumonisins cause pulmonary edema.

Multiple exposures to fumonisin cause most clinical signs, not a one-time acute dose. Mycotoxins in general are heat stable and there is no specific antidote to treat with. In the Kellerman study, clinical signs of nervousness, a wide-based stance, trembling, ataxia, reluctance to move, paresis of the lower lip and tongue, and the inability to eat occurred on day 8 post-administration of oral FB1.[13] Euthanasia was performed on day 10 post-administration when the horse was in a tetanic seizure. Neurologic signs progress to dementia, ataxia, agitation, hyperesthesia, and seizures. Horses may become stuporous, head press, and circle. Sudden death has been reported but typically clinical signs occur for several days before death.

There are no pathognomonic serum chemistry or complete blood count parameters to help diagnose ELEM, although the altered ratio of sphinganine to sphingosine (sphinganine:sphingosine[Sa:So] increases in serum or tissues) is helpful in a diagnosis but not readily available. Increased liver enzyme activities are detected in horses with neurologic and hepatotoxic forms of the disease. Characteristic gross lesions of ELEM in the central nervous system are described as malacia, degeneration, or liquefactive necrosis involving the subcortical white matter of one or both cerebral hemispheres. Necrotic lesions in the central nervous system lack cellular detail. The periphery of the lesion often is marked by perivascular hemorrhage and edema. Histologic lesions include centrilobular necrosis or hepatocyte vacuolization and fatty degeneration as well as centrilobular necrosis, bile stasis, and bile duct proliferation.

ELEM should be differentiated from other neurologic diseases that present as epizootics in horses. This includes equine herpesvirus 1 myeloencephalitis, botulism, Eastern and Western equine encephalitis, and Theiler's disease.

Most horses with ELEM die or are euthanized. Survivors often have residual neurologic deficits and never fully recover. Treatment is symptomatic and there is no antidote. Forages are the main diet for horses and there are fewer problems with mycotoxins in forages than in grain. Several studies have shown mycotoxins to be common in hay in Europe and the United States.[14]

Trichothecenes

Over 25% of global crop production is adversely affected by mycotoxins. Monogastrics are more susceptible to mycotoxicosis than ruminants, with the rumen more capable of detoxification of mycotoxins. Forages compose the largest portion of an equine diet, and there are typically fewer mycotoxins in forages than grains. *Aspergillus, Penicillium, Alternaria,* and *Fusarium* molds are involved in most of the mycotoxicosis in humans and animals. More than 500 mycotoxins have been identified that cause adverse effects in animals.[14] One of the major classes of mycotoxins posing serious hazards to humans and animals and potentially causing severe economic impact to the cereal industry is the trichothecenes, produced by many fungal genera.[15] The trichothecenes family contains more than 200 toxins of structurally related compounds produced by a broad range of species of fungi such as *Fusarium, Cephalosporium, Myrothecium, Trichoderma, Stachybotrys, Spicellum, Trichothecium,* and others in maize, oats, wheat, barley, rye, rice, fresh, dried fruits, grape juice, spices, and herbs.

In North America, the trichothecenes produced by *Fusarium* mainly contaminate cereal grains.

Vomitoxin (deoxynivalenol [DON]) is the most common trichothecene that causes adverse health effects in animals. Although T-2, HT-2, and 3- and 15-acetyldeoxynivalenol (3- and 15-ADON) are also involved with trichothecene mycotoxicosis. In wet, cool climates *Fusarium* mycotoxins can also affect the vegetative portion of the plant, the cob.[16] In these cases, the cobs need to be avoided and not fed to horses. Mycotoxin contamination can occur in hay, green feed, straw, and silage.

Trichothecenes causing adverse health in horses are divided into type A and B. Trichothecene mycotoxins contain a large number of compounds classified as tetracyclic sesquiterpenoids with a 12,13-epoxytrichothec-9-ene core structure.[16] Type A trichothecenes include T-2, HT-2, diacetoxyscirpenol (DAS), NX-2, and neosolaniol. Type B trichothecenes include deoxynivalenol, nivalenol, 3-ADON, 15-ADON, and deoxynivalenol-3-glucose. DON is the most common type B trichothecene, but 3- and 15-ADON can also be found. There are very few studies looking at the effects of 3- and 15- ADON in horses.

The main clinical signs of all trichothecene toxicosis are feed refusal, immunologic challenges, vomiting, skin dermatitis, and hemorrhage. The gastrointestinal system is the target of the trichothecenes. Diagnosis of trichothecene toxicosis is based on typical clinical signs and analytical identification of the trichothecene at elevated concentrations associated with causing adverse effects in that species. The lung may also be a target of trichothecenes. DON affected epithelial integrity of lung explants in both ex vivo and in vivo tissue culture systems.[17] The damage was observed histologically in the respiratory epithelium morphology and in resistance across the equine respiratory epithelial cells.

In a study looking at the association between forage mycotoxins and liver disease in horses, mycotoxins were found in 79% of the samples.[14] Ten mycotoxins were found on farms. These mycotoxins were fumonisin B1, 15-ADON, deoxynivalenol, zearalenone, aflatoxins B1 and G1, methylergonovine, nivalenol, verruculogen, and wortmannin.[14] Two cases of 29 contained DON and two cases contained 15-ADON.

In a study looking at the effects of feeding a blend of grains naturally contaminated with *Fusarium* mycotoxins on horses, 15 ppm DON and 0.8 ppm 15-AC DON were found in the grain.[18] Feed intake by all horses fed contaminated grains was reduced. Serum activities of γ-glutamyltransferase were higher in horses fed the diet containing contaminated grain compared with those fed the control diet on days 7 and 14 ($P = .047$ and .027, respectively), but not on day 21 ($P = .273$). Other hematology and serum chemistry measurements including serum immunoglobulin M(IgM), immunoglobulin G(IgG), and immunoglobulin A(IgA) were not affected by the diet.

A feeding trial using naturally contaminated oats with high (20.2 mg/kg) and low (0.49 mg/kg) levels of DON was conducted.[7] Daily DON intakes as high as 6.9 to 9.5 mg/100 kg bodyweight(BW) seem to have no major impact on the measured immune response of horses, indicating that this species has a high tolerance for DON.

T-2 and HT-2 toxins are in the group of Type A trichothecenes and may co-occur with another type A mycotoxin, DAS that causes similar clinical signs. Various *Fusarium, Stachybotrys,* and *Myrothecium* fungi can produce these toxins, including *Fusarium sporotrichioides, F acuminatum, F poae,* and *F langsethiae* that can infect crops and grasses in the field (eg, pasture grasses in cool, wet valleys) and particularly in unharvested overwinter cereal crops insulated with snow and hays stored in wet storage conditions. T-2 and HT-2 toxins can frequently be detected in oats, and processing oats can result in enrichment (an increase by up to 4 times in the oat byproducts) of T-2 and HT-2 toxins in the cleanings, small kernels and hull fraction, and a corresponding reduction in the de-hulled kernels by about 70% to 90%.[19] T-2 and HT-2 toxins often occur in field corn following hail damage in late summer, co-occurring with zearalenone and deoxynivalenol. T-2 toxin can be generated at temperatures between 0 °C and 32 °C (32–89.6 °F), with maximum synthesis occurring at less than 15 °C (<59 °F).[20]

HT-2 toxin can be naturally produced in plant material and is also the main metabolite of T-2 toxin. Similar to other trichothecene mycotoxins, T-2 and HT-2 toxins inhibit protein, DNA, and RNA synthesis, induce apoptosis and necrosis of cells, and cause lipid peroxidation. T-2 toxin is sometimes referred to as a "radiomimetic poison" causing similar clinical signs in animals as radiation. Clinical signs are typically feed refusal, weight loss, gastrointestinal damage with diarrhea and bloody diarrhea, skin lesions, neuroendocrine and liver changes, potential abortions, and altered immune responses. Lesions can involve local irritation, ulceration, and necrosis of the gastrointestinal tract and skin, damage to blood vessel walls with hemorrhagic diathesis, and cellular depletion of lymphoid organs.

Horses fed with a contaminated cereal, ranging from 0.5 to 204 mg T-2 toxin/kg or ppm, developed signs of locomotor alteration, pathologic changes were reported in the brain, liver, and kidney along with hepatic fatty degeneration, and several horses died a month postexposure.[21] In a long-term study, six mares were given a daily oral dose of 7 mg of purified T-2 toxin for 32 to 40 days with few adverse effects except skin lesions around the mouth in three mares.[22] The investigators reported no effects on the length of the inter-ovulatory interval, luteal and follicular phases, and fertilization. In several field cases, horses were fed wet stored hay containing 9 ppm (or mg/kg, dried weight basis) T-2 toxin with the horses developing colic, diarrhea and bloody diarrhea, and abortions (Mostrom MS. NDSU-VDL, toxicology section, mycotoxin results in 2009 to 2010, Fargo, ND). The US FDA does not have guidelines for T-2 and HT-2 toxins in animal feeds; however, the European Union recommendation on T-2 and HT-2 levels in complete feed in all species, except cats, is a maximum of 250 ppb or μg/kg or 0.25 ppm or mg/kg.[23] Similar to other trichothecene exposures, the treatment of T-2 and HT-2 toxin clinical signs is supportive care and switching to a "clean" feed.

Multiple mycotoxins can be present in feeds. Mycotoxins were evaluated in 122 samples from animal feeds in Tunisia during 2019.[24] Twenty-two mycotoxins were detected including aflatoxins, fumonisins, trichothecenes, deoxynivalenol, T-2 toxin, *Alternaria* toxins alternariol monomethyl ether, alternariol, tentoxin, along with ochratoxin A, enniatins, beauvericin, and zearalenone. Trichothecenes present in animal feeds were present in this order, DON > 15-ADON > 3-ADON > HT-2 >T-2 toxin > DAS.

Masked mycotoxins can be a concern when doing analysis for the parent compounds. Masked mycotoxins are parent compounds that are modified by plants as a defense mechanism. Detoxification processes of plants that are infected with the mold producing a mycotoxin are responsible for the conversion of the parent mycotoxin to mycotoxin derivatives, called masked mycotoxins. Masked mycotoxins are less toxic metabolites for plants according to their free forms. The parent mycotoxin and the masked mycotoxin have toxic effects on animals and humans. Masked mycotoxins are hydrolyzed into their free forms by human and animal intestinal microbiomes.

Zearalenone

Zearalenone is an estrogenic mycotoxin produced by numerous *Fusarium* species including *Fusarium graminearum, F culmorum, F equiseti, F sporotrichioides, and F moniliforme*. The fungi invade and produce zearalenone in corn, particularly corn stored on cobs in open bins, other cereal grains, hay, and straw. Environmental conditions of high humidity and moderate to lower temperatures will favor zearalenone production, particularly temperatures between less than 12 °C to 14 °C (53–57 °F) but can be produced at temperatures below freezing.

Zearalenone and its derivatives α- and β-zearalenol bind to estrogenic receptors (ERs), acting as a competitive agonist for ER-α and mixed agonist-antagonist for ER-β.[25] In the horse, the main conversion of zearalenone is to β-zearalenol with a lower amount of α-zearalenol, which is excreted in urine and feces, with the metabolites excreted in urine at approximately 100% glucuronide-conjugated forms.[26] Zearalenone can induce hyperestrogenism including enlargement of the uterus, swollen vulvas, rectal and vaginal prolapses, infertility with possible abnormal estrous cycles, early embryonic death, and possible abortions.

Natural zearalenone contamination at 2.7 ppm or mg/kg in the feed for horses was associated with feed refusal, enlarged edematous vulva, prolapsed vagina, enlarged uterus, and internal hemorrhage.[27] In a study of cycling trotter mares during the summer, purified zearalenone (in 1 mg/mL of ethyl alcohol) was given orally every day for a 10-day period starting 10 days after ovulation and continued until the subsequent ovulation.[28] The authors reported that (1) no effect on the length of the interovulatory intervals, luteal and follicular phases, (2) no significant influence was detected in plasma progesterone profiles, and (3) the follicular activity and uterine edema indicated no detectable adverse effect of zearalenone at a low dose on reproduction. Vance and colleagues studied the effect of chronic zearalenone exposure in cycling mares fed greater than 95% pure zearalenone at 0, 2, or 8 mg/day for three estrous cycles, followed by artificial insemination, and exposure through 16 days of pregnancy, or a total zearalenone exposure between 70 and 121 days.[29] The investigators reported no adverse uterine and ovarian effects, but pregnancy rates were mixed in mares on the low zearalenone exposure with only three maintaining pregnancy and fetal heartbeat by Day 30, compared with five of six control mares and all seven mares on the high zearalenone dose maintaining pregnancy. No significant changes were reported in the serum estradiol or progesterone levels for mares on zearalenone treatments compared with control mares; however, there was a significant increase in serum progesterone concentrations across the estrous cycles for the high zearalenone treated mares.[29] A study was reported by Minervini and colleagues of natural

Table 1
Mycotoxins that could cause adverse effects in equine but can be toxic to domestic animals[32,33]

Mycotoxin	Source	Clinical Effects	Diagnosis (Perform Analysis for Toxins in Feedstuffs)	Treatment
Citrinin	Aspergillus, Penicillium, Monascus in cereals	Tubular nephrosis Polydipsia/polyuria Azotemia Anorexia, emaciation	Clinical signs related to kidney damage and renal lesions. Often co-occurs with ochratoxin A in grain, do analytical testing in feed	Change feed and supportive care for renal failure
Dicoumarol	Penicillium, Aspergillus, Fusarium, Mucor, Humicolor in sweet clover (Melilotus spp) and sweet vernal grass (Anthoxanthum odoratum)	Interferes with regeneration of vitamin K1 and activation of prothrombin and factors VII, IX, X; subcutaneous, and organ hemorrhage, abortions, lameness, neurologic effects	Consuming moldy sweet clover hay, analysis of dicoumarol in hay at >10 to > 20 ppm can cause effects. Dicoumarol can remain toxic in hay for 3–4 years	Change to clean feed, vitamin K1 treatment for 5–7 days, and animals may need a whole blood or plasma transfusion
Ergot alkaloids	Claviceps purpurea in wheat, barley, rye, oats, triticale, and grasses (eg, brome, timothy, and quack grasses)	Peripheral gangrene (tail, feet, ears) and sloughing of tissue; suppressed prolactin secretion with agalactia at parturition	Clinical signs related to ergotism, may detect dark sclerotic bodies in cereals and grass seed heads, analysis for ergot alkaloids in cereal grain and grasses	Change to clean feed, supportive care for gangrene, and possible hoof damage or sloughing of hooves. Possible D2 receptor antagonism (eg, domperidone) for treatment of prolonged gestation in mares
Ochratoxin	Aspergillus, Penicillium in cereal grains, and cereal by-products, peanuts	Renal tubular nephrosis, hepatotoxic and immunosuppressive, teratogenic. Signs of anorexia, weight loss, polyuria/polydipsia. Ochratoxin can cross the placenta in equine and be detected in umbilical blood of foals[34]	The European Union recommends maximum 250 µg/g (ppb) for feed materials.[31] Perform analysis of ochratoxin A in feed. Clinical signs related to kidney and perhaps liver failure	Change feed and supportive care for organ failure

(continued on next page)

Table 1
(continued)

Mycotoxin	Source	Clinical Effects	Diagnosis (Perform Analysis for Toxins in Feedstuffs)	Treatment
Satratoxins	*Stachybotrys chartarum* in straws, forages reported in horses in Russia, Europe, South Africa	Oral ulcerations, salivation, and conjunctivitis progressing to leukopenia, agranulocytosis, thrombocytopenia, coagulopathy, and terminally fever, oral necrosis, hemorrhagic diarrhea, and death	Oral and gastrointestinal lesions, bone marrow hypoplasia, lymphoid depletion, mucosal hemorrhages. Fungal identification in forage, analytical testing for satratoxins G and H and roridin E in forages	
Slaframine "slobber factor"	*Rhizoctonia leguminicola* in red clover (*Trifolium* spp) and other legumes, "black patch" disease in forage. Swainsonine, a lysosomal storage disease from locoweed, can also be produced but not typically associated with this exposure, perhaps due to rapid dramatic effects and quick change of feed in animal	Quick onset of parasympathomimetic effects with excessive salivation and lacrimation, urination, diarrhea, anorexia, also can cause bradycardia and bradypnea. Other effects are weight loss, lower milk production, abortions	Clinical signs and detecting slaframine in forage. Hay storage may result in slaframine degradation over time (about 10% reduction in 10 months), but old hay may still cause slobbers for at least 2 years	Pre-administration of muscarinic antagonists, for example, atropine, block salivation but if atropine given after slaframine ingestion will not change adverse effects. After the slaframine source is removed from diet, signs usually dissipate within 4 days.
Tremorgens (Lolitrems A, B, C, D) Lolitrem B predominates	Drought or overgrazed perennial ryegrass (*Lolium perenne*) staggers caused by fungal endophyte *Epichloë festucae* var *lilii* Toxin is highest in seed. Lowest 2 cm of forage has high concentration of toxin	Clinical signs appear days after heavy dew or rainfall on forage. Signs start with head tremors, and muscle fasciculations of neck and legs, ataxia, dysmetria and legs stiffen lead to collapse and spasms followed by recovery. Death is rare, unless an accident occurs	Clinical signs and lesions are absent unless chronically affected animals that may have loss of Purkinje cells in the cerebellum. Mechanism of action may involve mycotoxin binding to brain gamma-aminobutyric acid receptors. Analysis for lolitrems is not readily available	Using minimal stress, remove animals from pasture or stop feeding hay. Provide a quiet, secure place for 3–7 days for recovery. No antidote known; activated charcoal may help but difficult to administer to excitable animals

Tremorgens (paspalitrems) Paspalinine, paspalitrem A, paspalitrems B	Paspalum staggers of dallis grass (Paspalum dilatatum) or bahia grass (Bahia oppositifolia) infested with the fungus Claviceps paspali that forms sclerotia. Occurs in warm, humid climates typically where dallis grass is grown	Mechanism of action is probable inhibition of gamma-aminobutyric acid. Clinical effects similar to lolitrems, but severity and clinical course generally less severe	Clinical signs and exposure to dallis grass. No lesions reported and analysis for paspalitrems not readily available	Remove animals from infected field and recovery will take 1–3 weeks. Mowing of pasture reduces exposure to sclerotia in the seeds and potential toxicosis in animals
Tremorgens (penitrem A)	Penicillium in corn, peanuts, and nuts	Tremors, incoordination, weakness can be stimulated with stress and exercise	Clinical signs and analysis for penitrem A in feed	Change feed, keep animal quiet with minimal stress; recovery within 7 days

exposure of male horses to zearalenone and subsequent evaluation of the in vitro effects of sperm cells to the urine zearalenone and its' derivatives concentrations on sperm chromatin structure stability.[30] The investigators found, after short-term exposure to zearalenone, α-zeararenol, and β-zearalenol at low-levels, a dose-related effect on sperm chromatin structure stability and genotoxic activity induced by zearalenone.

The US FDA does not have guidelines for zearalenone. Although the European Union does not have specific equine feed recommendations for maximum contamination of zearalenone, the general guidance levels for maximum zearalenone contamination range from 2000 μg/kg (ppb) for cereals and cereal products to 3000 μg/kg (ppb) for corn (maize) products.[31] There is no specific treatment for zearalenone exposure; generally, after stopping the exposure to zearalenone (unless very excessive) most animals will return to normal estrous cycling after 4 to 8 weeks.

SUMMARY

This article briefly covered mycotoxins occurring in feeds for equine. **Table 1** provides additional mycotoxins that equine may have exposure to in feeds and forages. As noted in the table, often little dose–response data are available for mycotoxins in the equine species and treatment for mycotoxicosis is supportive in clinical care.

As the analytical sensitivity improves, more mycotoxins will be identified. Correlating the mycotoxin with clinical signs will continue to be a clinical issue. Better interventions for mycotoxicosis are needed because they are a permanent part of animals' diets.

DISCLOSURE

The authors declare that there are no competing financial interests in the work described.

REFERENCES

1. Caloni F, Cortinovis C. Toxicological effects of aflatoxins in horses. Vet J 2011; 188(3):270–3.
2. Food and Drug Administration (FDA). Center for Veterinary Medicine. Office of Regulatory Affairs. Sec. 683.100 Action Levels for Aflatoxins in Animal Food, Compliance Policy Guide, March 2019. Rockville, MS. https://fda.gov.ICECI/ ComplianceManuals/CompliancePolicyGuidanceManual/default.htm. Accessed January 10, 2023.
3. Gunsen U, Yaroglu T. Aflatoxin in dog and horse feeds in turkey. Vet Hum Toxicol 2002;44(2):113–4.
4. Keller KM, Queiroz BD, Keller LAM, et al. The mycobiota and toxicity of equine feeds. Vet Res Commun 2007;31(8):1037–45.
5. Meerdink G. Mycotoxins. Clin Tech Equine Pract 2002;1:89–93.
6. Larsson P, Persson E, Tyden E, et al. Cell-specific activation of aflatoxin B1 correlates with presence of some cytochrome P450 enzymes in olfactory and respiratory tissues in horse. Res Vet Sci 2003;74(3):227–33.
7. Khol-Parisini A, Hellweg P, Razzazi-Fazeli E, et al. Highly deoxynivalenol contaminated oats and immune function in horses. Arch Anim Nutr 2012;66(2):149–61.
8. Butler T. Notes on a feeding experiment to produce leucoencephalitis in a horse, with positive results. J Comp Med Vet Arch 1902;23(8):498.

9. Wilson B, Maronpot P. Causative fungus agent of leucoencephalomalacia in equine animals. Vet Rec 1971;88(19):484–6.

10. Marasas WFO, Kellerman TS, Gelderblom WC, et al. Leukoencephalomalacia in a horse induced by fumonisin B₁ isolated from Fusarium moniliforme. Onderstepoort J Vet Res 1988;55(4):197–203.

11. Voss KA, Smith GW, Haschek WM. Fumonisins: Toxicokinetics, mechanism of action and toxicity. Anim Feed Sci Technol 2007;137(3–4):299–325.

12. Food and Drug Administration (FDA), Center for Veterinary Medicine. Guidance for Industry: Fumonisin Levels in Human Foods and Animal Feeds; Final Guidance, November 9, 2001 https://www.fda.gov/regulatory-information/search-fda-guidance-documents/guidance-industry-fumonisin-levels-human-foods-and-animal-feeds. Accessed January 10, 2023.

13. Kellerman TS, Marasas WF, Thiel PG, et al. Leukoencephalomalacia in two horses induced by oral dosing of fumonisin B₁. Onderstepoort J Vet Res 1990;57(4):269–75.

14. Durham AE. Association between forage mycotoxins and liver disease in horses. J Vet Intern Med 2022;36(4):1502–7.

15. Meneely J, Greer G, Kolawole O, et al. T-2 and HT-2 Toxins: Toxicity, occurrence and analysis: A review. Toxins 2023;15(8):481.

16. Mostrom M. Trichothecene toxicosis in animals. Rahway, NJ, Merck: Merck Veterinary Manual; 2022.

17. Van Cleemput J, Poelaert KCK, Laval K, et al. Deoxynivalenol, but not fumonisin B1, aflatoxin B1 or diesel exhaust particles disrupt integrity of the horse's respiratory epithelium and predispose it for equine herpesvirus type 1 infection. Vet Microbiol 2019;234:17–24.

18. Raymond SL, Smith TK, Swamy HV. Effects of feeding a blend of grains naturally contaminated with Fusarium mycotoxins on feed intake, metabolism, and indices of athletic performance of exercised horses. J Anim Sci 2005;83(6):1267–73.

19. Pettersson H, Nyman Jansson A, Lindberg JE. T-2 and HT-2 toxins in oats and the effects in horses. Utrecht, The Netherlands: Conference paper at Mykotoxin Workshop; 2008.

20. Zhang J, Liu X, Su Y, et al. An update on T-2 toxins: metabolism, immunotoxicity mechanism and human assessment exposure of intestinal microbiota. Heliuon 2022;8:e10012.

21. Gabal MA, Awad YL, Morcos MB, et al. Fusariotoxicoses of farm animals and mycotoxic leucoencepalomalacia of the equine associated with the finding of trichothecens in feedstuffs. Vet Hum Toxicol 1986;28(3):207–12.

22. Juhasz J, Nagy P, Huszenicza G, et al. Long-term exposure to T-2 fusarium mycotoxin fails to alter luteal function, follicular activity and embryo recovery in mares. Equine Vet J 1997;25:17–21.

23. Commission Recommendation of 27 March 2013 on the presence of T-2 and HT-2 toxins in cereals and cereal products. Off J Eur Union 2013;165. 12–5.

24. Juan C, Oueslati S, Manes J, et al. Multimycotoxin determination in Tunisian farm animal feed. J Food Sci 2019;84(12):3885–93.

25. Kuiper GG, Lemmen JG, Carlsson B, et al. Interaction of estrogenic chemicals and phytoestrogens with estrogen receptor beta. Endocrinology 1998;139:4252–63.

26. Songsermsakul P, Bohm J, Aurich C, et al. The levels of zearalenone and its metabolites in plasma, urine and faeces of horses fed with naturally, Fusarium toxin-contaminated oats. J Anim Physiol Anim Nutr 2013;97:155–61.

27. Gimeno A, Quintanilla JA. Analytical and mycological study of a natural outbreak of zearalenone mycotoxicosis in horses. Cairo, Egypt: Proceeding of the International Symposium of Mycotoxins; 1983. p. 387–92.

28. Juhasz J, Nagy P, Kulcsar M, et al. Effect of low-dose zearalenone exposure on luteal function, follicular activity and uterine oedema in cycling mares. Acta Vet Hung 2001;49(2):211–22.

29. Vance CK, Health King E, Bowers SD, et al. Reproductive performance of mares fed dietary zearalenone. Front Vet Sci 2019;6:423–34.

30. Minervini F, Lacalandra GM, Nicassio M, et al. Effects of in vitro exposure to natural levels of zearalenone and its derivatives on chromatin structure stability in equine spermatozoa. Theriogenology 2010;73:392–403.

31. Commission Recommendation (EU) 2016/1319 of 29 July 2016 amending Recommendation 2006/576/EC as regards deoxynivalenol, zearalenone and ochratoxin A in pet food (Textwith EEA relevance) Official J European Union 2016, L 208, p. 58-60.

32. Osweiler GD. Mycotoxins. Vet Clin North Am Equine Pract 2001;17(3):547–66.

33. Plumlee KH, Galey FD. Neurotoxic mycotoxins: A review of fungal toxins that cause neurological disease in large animals. J Vet Intern Med 1994;8:49–54.

34. Minervini F, Giannoccaro A, Nicassio M, et al. First evidence of placental transfer of ochratoxin A in horses. Toxins 2013;5:84–92.

Toxigenic Endophyte–Infected Tall Fescue and Ergot Alkaloids

Tim J. Evans, DVM, MS, PhD[a],*, Megan C. Romano, DVM[b]

KEYWORDS

- Agalactia • Dysgalactia • Dystocia • Ergopeptine alkaloids • Ergot alkaloids • Ergot
- Ergotism • Fescue toxicosis

KEY POINTS

- Equine ergopeptine alkaloid toxicosis (EEPAT) is caused by ergopeptine alkaloid (EPA) exposure in late-gestational mares and can be prevented by eliminating any exposure to EPAs at least 30 to 60 days before parturition and/or reversing hypoprolactinemia.
- In TE+ TFG, the endophyte, *Epichloë coenophiala*, lives within Continental tall fescue grass, *Lolium arundinaceum* (Schreb.) Darbysh), and produces EPAs, including ergovaline, the most abundant and arguably most toxic.
- EPAs (ergocornine, ergocristine, ergocryptine, ergosine, ergotamine, and, occasionally, ergovaline) are also produced by ergot fungus (*Claviceps purpurea*), which infects and replaces small grains and grass seeds with ergot bodies (sclerotia).
- In horses, EPAs are predominantly D_2-dopamine receptor agonists, suppressing prolactin secretion; prolactin is essential for normal equine mammary development, lactation, and other vital functions.
- EEPAT consistently presents at least as agalactia or dysgalactia in late-gestational mares and failure of passive transfer in foals; prolonged pregnancy, dystocia, and other reproductive abnormalities can also occur in mares, as can dysmaturity, overmaturity, postmaturity, and septicemia in foals.

INTRODUCTION

The corresponding author (TJE) has almost 30 years' experience diagnosing, treating, and researching the effects of "fescue toxicosis" and ergotism in livestock, hereinafter referred to as "ergopeptine alkaloid toxicosis" (EPAT). EPAT can have a devastating

[a] Department of Biomedical Sciences, College of Veterinary Medicine, University of Missouri-Columbia, W226 Veterinary Medicine Building, 1520 Rollins Street, Columbia, MO 65211, USA; [b] Department of Veterinary Science, Martin-Gatton College of Agriculture, Food, and Environment, University of Kentucky Veterinary Diagnostic Laboratory, 1490 Bull Lea Road, PO Box 14125, Lexington, KY 40512-4125, USA
* Corresponding author.
E-mail address: evanst@missouri.edu

Vet Clin Equine 40 (2024) 95–111
https://doi.org/10.1016/j.cveq.2024.01.001
0749-0739/24/© 2024 Elsevier Inc. All rights reserved.

impact on animal agriculture; however, negative outcomes can be mitigated by implementing modern agronomic/livestock management practices. This article reviews the origins, pathogenesis, and management of equine EPAT (EEPAT), particularly in late-gestational mares and their unborn/neonatal foals.

This review comprises 3 sections. The Introduction provides the rationale for continued interest in EPAT and reviews various mitigation approaches. The Discussion explains the roles of toxigenic endophyte–infected (TE+) tall fescue grass (TFG) (TE+ TFG); *Claviceps purpurea* (ergot)–infected grains/grasses; and ergot alkaloids (EAs), especially ergopeptine alkaloids (EPAs). The Summary/Clinical Care Points lists approaches to the diagnosis, treatment, and prevention of EEPAT in mares and foals. It is presumed throughout this review that other equine species respond to EPA exposure in the same way as horses.

History

The prevalence of Continental-genotype TFG in what is now called the "fescue belt" is the *initially intended* outcome of the University of Kentucky's discovery and development of the Kentucky-31 cultivar ("Suiter's grass") in the 1930s and its widespread distribution during the 1940s.[1–5] Kentucky-31 flourished where establishing pastures had been difficult, supporting the expansion of livestock production. By the late 1970s, it was recognized that most TFG within the United States was infected with *Epichloë coenophiala*.[1–3] Concurrently, awareness grew of a disease in Kentucky-31–exposed livestock, the clinical signs of which paralleled ergotism.[1,5]

Prevention attempts were made during the 1980s and 1990s to prevent "fescue toxicosis," by using endophyte-free TFG.[3–5] While no clinical signs occurred in exposed livestock, endophyte-free TFG grew poorly, with decreased stress/pathogen resistance (eg, drought, nematodes, insects, and others).[1,3,4] Alternative mitigation strategies were pursued that could still exploit the symbiosis between Kentucky-31 and its TE.[3,4] Research over the last 30 to 40 years has expanded understanding of the endophyte life cycle and the impacts of TFG/endophyte interactions on toxin production and accumulation and has fostered the development of management practices designed to decrease EPA exposure in animals consuming TE+ TFG.[1–4,6,7] Genetic modification has been used to infect improved TFG varieties with various nontoxic/less toxic endophytes, and multiple "safe" endophyte-infected (E+) tall fescue varieties are now commercially available.[4,6,7]

From "Fescue Toxicosis" and Reproductive Ergotism to Ergopeptine Alkaloid Toxicosis

Other mitigation strategies have attempted to discover the ultimate toxicants responsible for "fescue toxicosis."[1] Administration of these compounds could serve as a model to test efficacy of therapeutic approaches and accuracy of diagnostic tests. The debate continues about which toxin(s) ultimately participates in receptor-mediated interactions and cause clinical signs in ruminants, primarily because dosages of TE+ TFG seeds or pastures, defined in terms of ergovaline concentrations, might not reflect the exposure dosage of the ultimate toxicant.[1,8,9] However, breakdown products/metabolites often cause clinical signs of intoxication (eg, aflatoxins), and oral exposure dosages are still defined in terms of the parent compounds. In horses, the consensus is that EPAs are ultimately responsible for causing both "fescue toxicosis" and "reproductive ergotism" in horses.[1,10,11] The semisynthetic EPA, bromocriptine, has effectively replicated "fescue toxicosis" in a pony model and was subsequently used to demonstrate efficacy of domperidone for mitigating the associated agalactia and prolonged gestation.[10,12–14] Additionally, EPAs are potent

D_2-dopamine receptor (D_2DR) agonists, whether or not their breakdown products/metabolites also play a role. Furthermore, measured dietary concentrations of EPAs, especially ergovaline, reliably predict the development of clinical signs in mares and foals.[1,10,11,15]

In horses, there are multiple advantages to focusing on total EPA concentrations. Collectively referring to "fescue toxicosis" and "reproductive ergotism" as EEPAT highlights 2 clinical realities. Firstly, EPA-induced hypoprolactinemia and subsequent agalactia/dysgalactia in late-gestational mares is not limited to the "fescue belt."[1,10,11,16] Secondly, total dietary EPA concentrations reflect potential contributions from multiple sources. Agalactia/dysgalactia in a late-gestational mare should immediately raise concerns about EPAs, regardless of where that mare is located. Early recognition can facilitate removal of contaminated feed and/or treatment of mares, increasing chances of foal survival, especially with particularly susceptible mares.[1,10,11]

DISCUSSION
The Role of Toxigenic Endophyte–Infected Continental Tall Fescue Grass
Continental genotype of tall fescue grass
TFG is referred to as *Lolium arundinaceum* (Schreb.) Darbysh, *Schnedonorus arundinaceus* (Schreb.) Dumont, and *Festuca arundinacea* (Schreb), often with only the italicized binomials written (**Fig. 1**).[1–5,11,16] The TFG predominantly discussed herein, especially Kentucky-31, originated from the Continental genotype and is a perennial cool-season, summer-active grass.[2–5] It represents the primary forage for an estimated greater than 8.5 million cattle and 700,000 horses in North America, causing production losses approaching $2 billion/year.[1,4,5,11,16] TFG reportedly grew on greater than 35 million acres in the upper Southeastern and lower Midwestern United States (the "fescue belt"/"fescue suitability zone").[1–5,9,16] States comprising the "fescue belt" include Missouri*, Kansas, Oklahoma, Arkansas*, Tennessee*, Mississippi, Alabama, Georgia, South Carolina*, North Carolina*, Virginia*, Maryland,

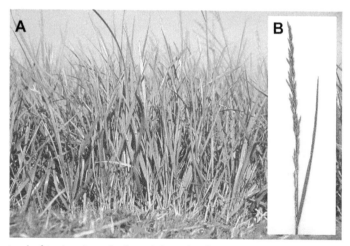

Fig. 1. A stand of toxigenic endophyte–infected *Lolium arundinaceum* (Schreb.) Darbysh), including both vegetative and reproductive tillers (*A*). Each tiller comprises roots and leaves. Vegetative tillers are primarily leaves; reproductive tillers produce a stem, seed heads, roots, and leaves (*B*). (Both images courtesy Drs. Robert Kallenbach and Greg Bishop-Hurley, University of Missouri.)

Pennsylvania, West Virginia*, Ohio*, Kentucky*, Indiana*, and Illinois*, (*indicates>50% of state within the "fescue belt").[1,11,15,16]

Toxigenic tall fescue endophyte

Continental TFG contains multiple potentially toxic xenobiotics; pyrrolizidine alkaloids (eg, loline, N-formyl loline, and N-acetyl loline) and the diphenanthrene alkaloids perloline and perlolidine have been reported in both endophyte-free and TE+ TFG. However, these and other compounds are considered minor contributors to the hardiness of some TFG varieties or the pathogenesis of TFG-related toxidromes observed in the United States.[1,11]

It is generally accepted that TFG/TE interactions are essential for the survivability of Kentucky-31 under adverse conditions and the etiology of its associated disease syndromes.[1-5,11,16] The TFG endophyte is referred to as *Epichloë coenophiala, Neotyphodium coenophialum, Acremonium coenophialum,* and *E typhina*; it infects ≥90% of TFG within the "fescue belt."[1-7,11,16] *E coenophiala (N coenophialum)* grows within the intercellular spaces of leaf sheaths, stems, and caryopses/seeds (traditionally highest concentrations) of Kentucky-31, producing various secondary metabolites, including ergovaline and other ergot alkaloids (EAs)[1-5,11,15,16] (**Fig. 2**). While concentrations are reportedly highest in TE+ TFG seed heads, ergovaline is found in other parts of the plant, and recent research suggests that the highest concentrations may actually be present in the bottom 2 inches (5 cm).[1,11,17] Ergovaline concentrations generally range between 0.2 and 0.6 mg/kg (ppm) in TE+ TFG (>1 mg/kg (ppm) in seed heads).[1,4,5,11,17]

Ergotized Small Grains/Grasses

Ergotism (reproductive, gangrenous, hyperthermic, and nervous/convulsive forms) represents an ancient disease affecting both humans and animals—St. Anthony's fire, the Salem witch trials, the French revolution, and the psychedelic drug lysergic acid diethylamide.[10,11,16,18] The EPAs ergotamine, ergocristine, ergosine, ergocornine, and ergocryptine predominate within the black/dark brown/purple ergot bodies (sclerotia) of *Claviceps purpurea*.[10,11,15,18] Unlike endophytes, sclerotia are externally visible, replacing individual seeds in seed heads of small cereal grains (eg, oats,

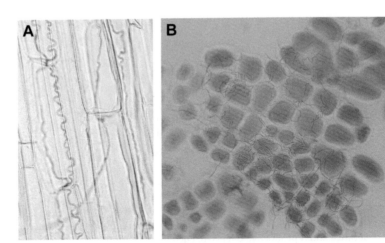

Fig. 2. Fungal hyphae of the toxigenic tall fescue endophyte, *Epichloë coenophiala*, stained with aniline blue, appear as "squiggly" linear structures within tall fescue tillers (*A*) and seed (*B*), respectively. (Both images courtesy Dr. Carolyn Young, North Carolina State University.)

barley, wheat, and especially rye and triticale) and common pasture grasses, including TE+ TFG (**Fig. 3**), bluegrasses, bentgrasses and redtops, bromegrasses, canary grasses, cocksfoot and orchard grasses, June grasses, love grasses, quackgrasses and wheatgrasses, ryegrasses, timothy, and wild barleys, oats, and ryes.[10,11] Germination and growth is facilitated by cool, wet springs in the Northwestern United States and the northern Great Plains.[4,10,11,15,18] Horses are most often exposed to ergot in contaminated pastures or hays, processed (especially pelletized) feeds, or screenings from ergotized grains.[10,11,15,18] The total EPA concentration within an individual sclerotium ranges from 2000 to 10,000 mg/kg (ppm).[10,11]

Ergot Alkaloids/Ergopeptides

Classification and structure

EAs are a complex class of compounds with at least 3 systems of nomenclature. Most naturally occurring EAs are isolated from fungi in the *Epichloë* (*Neotyphodium*) and *Claviceps* genera.[1–4,7,10,11,16] In 1 system, EAs are divided into clavines, lysergic acid, simple lysergic acid amides, and ergopeptides or EPAs.[7] EPAs are tetrapeptides comprising lysergic acid and 3 amino acids. Ergovaline is primarily of TE+ TFG origin.[1–3,10,11,16] The predominant EPAs associated with *C purpurea* include ergocornine, ergocryptine, ergocristine, ergosine, and ergotamine (**Fig. 4**).[10,11,15,16,18]

Mechanisms of action

Hypoprolactinemia: reproductive effects. Dopamine inhibits prolactin secretion by lactotropes in the anterior pituitary gland, or adenohypophysis.[1,10] Because EPAs,

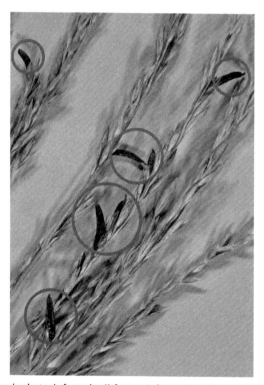

Fig. 3. Toxigenic endophyte–infected tall fescue infected by *Claviceps purpurea*; ergot sclerotia circled. (Image courtesy Dr. Tim Evans and Karen Clifford, University of Missouri.)

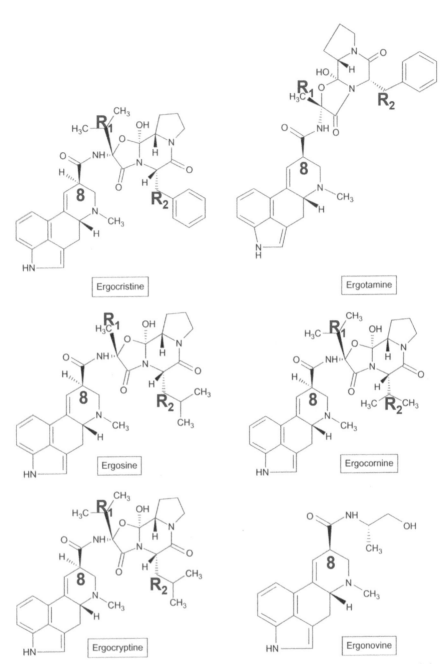

Fig. 4. The 5 predominant ergopeptine alkaloids produced by *Claviceps purpurea,* and the simple lysergic amide, ergonovine/ergometrine. The "8" denotes the C-8 carbon, around which epimerization to the ergopeptinine alkaloids occurs. "R_1" and "R_2" denote functional groups. R_1 is either an isopropyl group (ie, ergocornine, ergocristine, and α-ergocryptine) or a methyl group (ie, ergosine and ergotamine). R_2 can be methyl benzyl (ie, ergocristine and ergotamine), isopropyl (ie, ergocornine), or isobutyl (ie, α-ergocryptine and α-ergosine). Regarding ergovaline, R_1 is a methyl group; R_2 is an isopropyl group.[18]

especially ergovaline and ergotamine, are potent D_2DR agonists, hypoprolactinemia is the hallmark endocrine disruptive effect in late-gestational mares.[1,10,11] Normal lactation in mares is exquisitely dependent on prolactin secretion, unlike cattle. EPAs mimic dopamine's agonism of D_2DRs in lactotropes, producing hypoprolactinemia and agalactia/dysgalactia, especially in mares in late gestation.[1,10,11,15,16,18,19] Prolactin functions in the endocrine regulation of other physiologic processes in pregnant mares, including steroidogenesis during pregnancy and the onset of parturition.[11,19] Prolonged gestation in EPA-exposed mares likely depends on hypoprolactinemia-induced alterations in uterofetoplacental steroid metabolism or inhibition of corticotropes in the fetal anterior pituitary.[1,10,11,15,19] Bromocriptine administered to late-gestational pony mares suppresses serum prolactin concentrations and prevents the increase in progestins or progestogens during the last 30 days of gestation **(Fig. 5)**.[12–14] Signs of impending parturition, for example, rapid increase in udder development, accumulation of colostrum at teat orifices ("waxing"), and increased calcium concentration in mammary secretions are often absent/minimal with hypoprolactinemia.[1,10,11,13,14] Without such indicators, delivery is frequently unexpected/unattended, contributing to foal morbidity and mortality.[1,10,11,14]

Vasoconstriction: gangrenous and hyperthermic effects. EPA-induced vasoconstriction occurs due to the inhibition of D_1-dopaminergic receptors and partial α_1-adrenergic and serotonin receptor agonism.[1–5] Clinical signs arising from vasoconstriction (eg, hyperthermia, dry gangrene, and necrotic fat) characterize bovine "fescue toxicosis"; abortion and altered placental function are also possible.[1,4,5,10,11,20–23] At lower EPA concentrations generally found in TE+ TFG, the magnitude of clinical signs largely depends on ambient environmental temperatures.[1,10] The much higher concentrations in ergot can result in effects being less dependent on ambient temperature (eg, necrotic tail switches of cattle during spring or summer).[1,10,11]

While reproductive effects of EPAs predominate in horses, especially pregnant mares, administration of TE+ TFG seeds resulted in vasoconstriction of the medial palmar artery; the vasoactive abilities of various EAs, especially EPAs, were confirmed in vitro.[20,21] One aggregate risk study identified TE+ TFG exposure as a laminitis risk factor.[24] Other studies indicate adverse effects on thermoregulatory mechanisms in exercised TE+ TFG–exposed horses.[22,23] Minimizing exposure of individuals predisposed to laminitis or high-performing athletes, particularly those performing in high ambient temperatures, is advisable.

Ligand/receptor interactions. Decreased feed intake, and altered gut motility and nutrient absorption, particularly in cattle, may be associated with interactions between EPAs (and perhaps other EAs) and D_1, D_2, and/or other dopaminergic receptor types.[1,2,10] Impaired adaptations to seasonal photoperiod changes have occurred in mares exposed to TE+ TFG; this may be mediated by neurotransmitter imbalance within the pituitary and pineal glands and may involve interactions between EAs and norepinephrine, epinephrine, dopamine, serotonin, and melatonin receptors.[1,10,25] Hypothyroidism has occurred in EPA-exposed foals, with enlarged thyroid glands characterized by distended thyroid follicles. The pathogenesis remains uncertain.[1,11,15]

Reproductive Aspects

Clinical signs in late-gestation mares and foals
Lactational abnormalities and failure of passive transfer. Clinical signs in pregnant mares and their foals include agalactia/dysgalactia in mares, even in the absence of other clinical signs, and failure of passive transfer (FPT) in foals.[1,10–16,18,19] Less

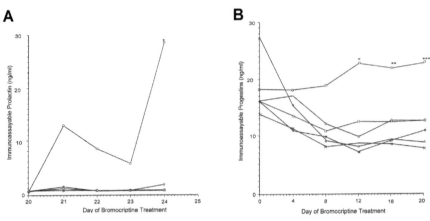

Fig. 5. Effects of bromocriptine (semisynthetic ergopeptine alkaloid) on circulating concentrations of immunoassayable prolactin (*A*) and progestins or progestogens (*B*) in late-gestational pony mares. Open circles represent negative controls; all other lines depict bromocriptine-treated groups. Decreases in prolactin and progestin/progestogen concentrations are typical of what is observed in late-gestational mares exposed to ergopeptine alkaloid–contaminated grains, pastures, or hay. Bromocriptine treatment began on day 300 of gestation and continued until after foaling. Asterisks denote statistically significant concentration differences (*P < .05, **P < .01, and***P < .001, respectively) between treatment groups and negative controls.[11,13,14]

frequently, generally at higher EPA concentrations, effects can include prolonged gestation, dystocia, premature placental separation, placental thickening/edema, retained fetal membranes, and/or metritis.[1,10,11,15,18,19] Severe clinical signs in fetuses/neonates, including fetal asphyxia, abortion, stillbirth, weakness, dysmaturity/over-maturity, septicemia, and neonatal mortality, occur most frequently when mares exhibit other clinical signs besides lactational abnormalities.[1,10,11,15,19] Clinically significant dietary EPA concentrations in regards to lactational abnormalities/FPT are likely to be $\geq$200 µg/kg (ppb) or 0.20 mg/kg (ppm), on a dry-weight basis; however, no minimal toxic concentrations have been established for mares.[15] Although some references suggest that some populations of mares can consume EPA concentrations $\leq$0.3 mg/kg (ppm) with minimal risk, concentrations of EPAs, especially ergovaline, $\geq$0.05 mg/kg have been associated with agalactia/dysgalactia in individual mares.[1–5,11,15] Occasional clinical cases have occurred in mares consuming fescue hay with $\geq$0.1 mg/kg ergovaline.[1,10,11] Agalactia/dysgalactia have occurred in multiple mares at 0.5 to 1.5 mg/kg total EPAs; some individuals anecdotally developed agalactia/dysgalactia at ergotamine concentrations as low as 0.05 mg/kg[10,11] Due to the sensitivity of late-gestational mares, the author's recommendation is to maintain EPA concentrations less than 0.025 mg/kg (ppm) if possible.[1,10]

Prolonged gestation, foal dysmaturity/overmaturity/postmaturity, and dystocia. Despite suboptimal placental function and fetal growth conditions, fetuses frequently continue growing during the prolonged gestation in EPA-exposed mares.[1,10] Foals are often described, depending on the reference and specific clinical presentation, as dysmature/overmature/postmaturity—frequently large and gangly, often with long, fine haircoats, poor muscle mass and suckling reflex, overgrown hooves without eponychium, and, possibly, prematurely erupted central incisors.[1,10,11,15] Thyroid pathology might contribute to these abnormalities.[1,10,11,15]

Parturition is normally initiated by the foal, requiring appropriate fetal presentation, position, and posture; foal dysmaturity/overmaturity/postmaturity and increased size likely contributes to the incidence of dystocias in EPA-exposed mares.[1,10,11,13–15] Foaling difficulties are often associated with retained fetal membranes and metritis (mares), FPT and septicemia (foals), and trauma during delivery, including death (both mares and foals).[1,10,11,15]

Abortion/stillbirth. EPA-induced abortions and stillbirths are less common than prolonged gestation.[1,5,11,15,19] Abortions appear more common with higher EPA doses produced by *C purpurea*; bromocriptine administration caused abortion in a pony model.[1,10,11,13–15] Additionally, ergot sclerotia can contain ergonovine (see **Fig. 4**), a simple lysergic acid/ergoline alkaloid/carboxamide.[7,10] Along with inhibiting prolactin secretion and causing vasoconstriction, ergonovine also stimulates myometrial smooth muscle contraction.[7,10,11]

Clinical signs in nonpregnant/early gestational mares
Impaired adaptations to seasonal photoperiod changes have occurred in TE+ TFG–exposed mares. The prolonged spring transitional period might be mediated by neurotransmitter imbalance within the pituitary and pineal glands and, possibly, interactions between EPAs and dopaminergic, serotonergic, and other receptors.[1,10,11,25] Under these circumstances, clusters of small-sized to medium-sized ovarian follicles and irregular or prolonged estrus without ovulation are not uncommon.[1,10,11,15,25] Embryonic death has been reportedly associated with EPA exposure early in pregnancy. Short-term, experimental exposures to low EA concentrations, including EPAs, between days 65 to 100 of gestation, have altered catecholamine metabolism, even when prolactin concentrations did not differ between treatment groups.[1,10,11,16] Therefore, potential EPA sources should be withdrawn from the diet of mares with abnormalities in seasonal cyclicity, early embryonic loss, and/or other reproductive abnormalities; mares bred with cooled-extended or frozen semen; and embryo transfer donor and recipient mares.[1,10,11]

Clinical signs in stallions
EPA-induced hypoprolactinemia is associated with reduced libido in rams and decreased gonadal and accessory sex gland weights in rodents. Otherwise, little data exist regarding the effects of receptor-mediated, EPA exposure on male fertility.[1,10] In ruminants, both males and females are susceptible to hyperthermic effects of EAs on reproduction. Similar effects have not been demonstrated in stallions; however, 1 study evaluating effects of TE+ TFG seeds on stallions and yearling colts demonstrated minimal adverse effects in the stallions, but possible heat stress–related effects on the colts.[1,10,19,26–28] Although there is currently insufficient evidence to suggest additional precautions in colts or breeding stallions exposed to low dietary EPA concentrations, when there is concern about a stallion's fertility, or where valuable prepubertal colts will experience high ambient temperatures, eliminating EPA exposure is reasonable, especially if measures are already in place for mares.[1,10,19,26,27]

Other Relevant Information

Toxicokinetics
Over the last 25 years, there have been few additions to the literature concerning EPA toxicokinetics in livestock, reflecting the complexities of these compounds and possible analytical challenges of accurately measuring EPAs in certain matrices. In nonruminants, intestinal EPA absorption possibly involves active transport, and hepatic metabolism and excretion appear to be dependent on molecular weight.[1,10] Larger

EPAs (>450 Da) likely undergo primary biliary excretion; smaller alkaloids (<350 Da) are generally excreted in urine, with or without additional hepatic metabolism.[1,10,29] In cattle, although the effects may persist longer, intravenously administered EPAs are rapidly cleared from the blood.[1,10] There is speculation that ergovaline is broken down in the rumen into lysergic acid, lysergol, and simple lysergic acid amides (collectively "ergoline alkaloids").[1,9,10,29] These compounds may be more efficiently absorbed than ergovaline.[1,8,9] Urinary excretion occurs rapidly in ruminants; urinary EA concentrations increase or decrease accordingly within 12 hours of introduction or withdrawal from TE+ TFG pastures.[29] Newer analytical methods are potentially better able to elucidate EPA disposition and toxicokinetics in livestock.[30,31]

Relative toxicity
Relative EPA activities have been assessed using in vitro models. Unfortunately, results can vary widely, with variables including receptor interactions assessed; species of origin for cells/tissues; types of cells/tissue location; availability, purity, and stability of the toxins evaluated; and others. Ergovaline and ergotamine reportedly have similar activities; corresponding activities of other EPAs are usually orders of magnitude less.[1,10,21]

Ergopeptine alkaloid/ergopeptinine epimerization
The EPAs discussed herein (ie, ergovaline, ergocornine, ergocristine, ergocryptine, ergosine, and ergotamine) can undergo epimerization at C-8, converting into the corresponding ergopeptinine (ie, ergovalinine, ergocorninine, ergocristinine, ergocryptinine, ergosinine, and ergotaminine).[30] The circumstances of epimerization/conversion are poorly understood and have been considered a laboratory phenomenon.[30,31] Until recently, EPAs (R epimers) were considered the active forms; ergopeptinine isomers (S epimers) were considered inactive or less active.[30–33] The EPA concentrations discussed herein were measured using high-performance liquid chromatography (HPLC)-fluorescence.[1,10,34,35] More sensitive analytical methods, using ultra HPLC-tandem mass spectrometry, can measure concentrations of both isomers in feedstuffs and, potentially, biological matrices.[30–33] Experimental dietary EPA exposure doses are now commonly expressed in terms of total ergopeptine and ergopeptinine concentrations.[20]

Differences in individual susceptibility
Hypoprolactinemic effects of EPAs depend on dopaminergic receptor–mediated interactions.[1,10,11] Individual mares differ in susceptibility, possibly due to variation in the number of receptors available for EPA binding. Additionally, single-nucleotide polymorphisms in these receptors and other target molecules might produce increased or decreased tolerance of individuals to EPAs, as is reported in cattle.[36,37] Another recent cattle research demonstrated potential breed differences in susceptibility and individual animal traits/potential biomarkers for increased sensitivity within a population.[38] Finally, in ruminants, some animals apparently adapt over time to TE+ TFG exposure, with naïve animals more likely to exhibit adverse health effects.[39,40]

Effects on placental development and fetal growth in sheep
Recent articles have evaluated dietary EA effects on placental development, fetal growth, and birthweight in pregnant, EA-naïve ewes; exposure caused intrauterine growth restriction (IUGR).[39,40] Despite species differences in reproductive physiology and pathophysiological responses to EAs, and, more specifically, EPAs, the dysmaturity/overmaturity/postmaturity in foals born to EPA-exposed mares likely reflects aspects of the IUGR observed in this ovine model.[1,10,11,15,39,40]

Novel endophyte–infected Mediterranean tall fescue grass and equine fescue edema/ edema syndrome

Especially in Australia and New Zealand, AR542 (MaxP or MaxQ) E + Mediterranean genotype of TFG (MGTFG) has been associated with a suspected toxic syndrome, equine fescue edema (EFO).[41,42] The MGTFG or summer-dormant genotype enters a semidormant phase during hot dry summers, resurging in fall and winter.[41–43] During its autumn resurgence, the MGTFG has exceptional growth; however, it is better suited for warmer, drier climates due to failure to survive prolonged freezing periods.[43] The pathogenesis of EFO apparently depends on infection by a novel endophyte, either the AR542 (MaxP or MaxQ) or AR584 (MaxQII) form of *E coenophiala*.[41–43] While the definitive ultimate toxicants remain disputed, clinical signs of EFO include anorexia, lethargy, and subcutaneous edema of the head, neck, thorax, and abdomen, apparently associated with hypoproteinemia, particularly hypoalbuminemia.[41,42] Most affected animals survive, although fatalities have occurred. Pathologically, gastrointestinal (GI) edema accompanied eosinophilic infiltration but not necrosis.[44]

SUMMARY/CLINICS CARE POINTS
Management of Equine Ergopeptine Alkaloid Toxicosis in Late-Gestational Mares

Diagnosis
Clinical signs

- Lack of mammary development and agalactia/dysgalactia are sometimes the only signs.[1,10,11,15,18]
- Unexpected parturition without mammary development and "waxing"
- Prolonged gestation; especially ≥360 days
- "Red bag" presentation: premature placental separation of chorioallantois, preceding foal passage through the birth canal; retained, potentially thickened fetal membranes; and/or metritis
- Dystocia, larger-than-normal foal, possible malposition, foal's neck frequently reflected sideways
- Frequent FPT; increased susceptibility to septicemia
- Weak, "overmature", "dummy" foal; incoordination and poor suckling reflex; possible hypothyroidism
- Occasional abortion or stillbirth

Bloodwork

- Mare or foal—possible stress leukogram from prolonged parturition/dystocia; abnormal leukogram caused by septicemia[1,10,11,15]
- Mares—decreased serum prolactin and progestogen concentrations (measured as progesterone by radioimmunoassay) during the last 30 days of gestation (see **Fig. 5**); increased serum estradiol-17β reported
- Foals—decreased serum triiodothyronine, plasma adrenocorticotropin hormone, and cortisol concentrations

Ultrasonography

- Thickened placenta and large foal[1,15]

Pathology

- Thickened, edematous fetal membranes ("placenta") without significant bacterial growth; most severe in chorioallantois near the cervical star; amnion edematous throughout; umbilical cord possibly edematous[1,15,19]
- Fetal membranes ruptured in the uterine body

- Foals abnormally large; overgrown hooves (increased growth of eponychium); variable incisor eruption, including premature eruption
- Enlarged thyroid glands in foals (not apparent grossly); microscopically, large, distended follicles lined by flattened cuboidal epithelium
- Uterine rupture, metritis, and peritonitis post-dystocia

Forage diagnostics
- Few differentials for agalactia/dysgalactia; investigating potential EPA sources critical, especially if multiple mares affected[1,3,10,11,15]
- Identify all potential EPA sources, including TFG and ergot in pastures, hays, and/or grains.
- Analyze forage for total concentrations of ergovaline, ergocornine, ergocristine, ergocryptine, ergosine, and ergotamine ± the corresponding ergopeptinines, plus ergonovine and ergonovinine
- Analyze feeds containing small grains (eg, barley, oats, and wheat), especially pelleted products, for the aforementioned EPAs
  - Relevant ergovaline/ergotamine concentrations
    - less than 0.025 ppm, ideal total EPA concentrations via HPLC-fluorescence
    - ≥0.05 ppm: agalactia/dysgalactia in an individual mare
    - ≥0.10 ppm: agalactia/dysgalactia in multiple mares ± more severe effects
    - ≥0.30 ppm: agalactia/dysgalactia and more severe effects in multiple mares
- *E coenophiala* not visible externally; detection requires microscopy/special staining, monoclonal antibody enzyme-linked immunosorbent assay
- Toxigenic endophyte detection not useful; greater than 90% TFG in the "fescue belt" likely infected

Treatment
General
- Owner suspects premature placental separation: confirm with veterinarian/follow instructions to deliver foal[1,10,15]
- Dystocia: immediate veterinary intervention (potentially C-section), follow-up care for metritis, vaginal trauma, and/or adhesions
- Symptomatic/supportive care as needed for prolonged gestation, retained fetal membranes, and/or laminitis in mares; septicemia, joint infections, and/or angular limb deformities in foals; other problems
- Remove postpartum mares from TE+ TFG for 5 to 15 days or longer, until the mare is lactating well
  - ± milk replacer/nurse mare

Domperidone
- D_2-dopamine receptor antagonist[1,10,11,15,19,45]
- Physiologic antidote for agalactia/dysgalactia
  - Indications as per the package insert for Equidone gel, a commercially available product containing domperidone
    - Agalactia/dysgalactia prior to foaling: 1.1 mg/kg by mouth every 24 hours for 10 to 15 days before due date; continue up to 5 to 15 days after foaling until the mare is lactating well (**Fig. 6**)
    - Confirmed prolonged gestation ≥360 days: as earlier; especially if no mammary development (see **Fig. 6**)
    - Agalactia post-foaling: 1.1 mg/kg by mouth every 12 hours for ≥2 days (until lactating); continued at 1.1 mg/kg by mouth every 24 hours for ≥3 more days (up to 15 days after foaling)

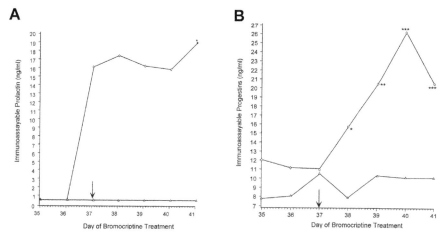

Fig. 6. Decreased circulating concentrations of immunoassayable prolactin (*A*) and progestins or progestogens (*B*) rapidly increased after the initiation of domperidone therapy (*open diamonds*) in bromocriptine-treated pony mares. No significant alterations in these parameters were observed in bromocriptine-treated mares following reserpine treatment (*open triangles*). Domperidone or reserpine administration began on day 337 of gestation. Asterisks denote statistically significant differences (*$*P<.05$, $**P<.01$, and $***P<.001$, respectively) between treatments.[11,13,14]

- Other usage is off-label, but could be indicated
- ○ Precautions/interactions
  - As per the package insert for Equidone gel, premature parturition, low birth weight, and foal morbidity or mortality possible with administration greater than 15 days before due date
  - Colostrum leaking and elevated calcium possible; elevated calcium concentrations no longer predict impending foaling
    - Can reduce to one-half dose every 12 hours; if loss continues, one-half dose every 24 hours; further as needed
    - Save colostrum; monitor foal's serum immunoglobulin (Ig) G
  - Domperidone stimulates GI motility; avoid in mares with GI blockage or perforation
  - May affect reproductive hormone concentrations in humans; pregnant and lactating women should handle domperidone-containing products with extreme caution; safety in lactating women and their nursing children not evaluated; consult a physician in case of exposure
  - Especially in humans, domperidone metabolism is inhibited when administered concurrently with some drugs, including erythromycin and ketoconazole; causes multifold increase in exposure dose

Other treatments
- Foal:[1,10,15]
  - ○ Banked colostrum
  - ○ Serum IgG monitoring
    - ± plasma tranfusion
  - ○ ± Antibiotics for septicemia
- Mare:[1,10,15]
  - ○ Retained fetal membranes, premature placental separation, and/or dystocia

- Oxytocin: 10 to 20 IU intramuscular, intravenous, or subcutaneous every 2 to 3 hours (higher dosages are recommended by some references)
- Uterine infusion (fluids, other therapies)
- ± Antibiotics/anti-inflammatories, as indicated

Alternative drugs
- "Binders" marketed to prevent ergovaline absorption; efficacy unknown; cross-reaction with other EPAs/EAs unknown[1,10,12–15]
- Reserpine, perphenazine, and other medications for treating/preventing agalactia and other clinical signs in horses; much less effective than domperidone

Prevention
- Far better than treatment[1,10,15,19,45]
- While not all are essential, practical, and/or affordable in all situations, incorporating the following should help minimize risk

Client communication
- Early discussion with owners of mares foaling in "fescue belt"[1,10,11,15,45]
  - What to look for; when to contact veterinarian
    - Mammary development/signs of impending parturition
      - Domperidone administration prevents using mammary development/calcium concentration of mammary secretions for predicting impending parturition
    - Parturition not progressing, lactation less than expected, fetal membranes retained, and/or the foal is abnormal
      - Have them call immediately, if there are any questions.
    - Mares and foals should be examined within 12 hours after parturition, especially if concerns about lactational abnormalities or foal's nursing ability

Animal management
- Remove mares from possible EA sources (TE+ TFG pastures/hay and ergotized grains/grasses) before late gestation[1,10,11,15,45]
  - 90 days before foaling is ideal; not always feasible; consider in mares with history of "fescue toxicosis," abortion, stillbirth, and/or dystocia
  - No mares should be exposed to sources of EPAs/other EAs beyond day 300
  - Good breeding records, including serial pregnancy examinations with ultrasound in early gestation help determine when to remove mares from EPA sources; especially if removal cannot occur prior to day 300
  - Recommend removal from TE+ TFG 40 to 60 days before foaling, if breeding history/pregnancy examination records are incomplete
- If removal from TE+ TFG is not possible, administer domperidone (see *Treatment*)

Forage management
- Identify and analyze potential EPA sources (see Forage Diagnostics section)[1,3,4,10,11,15,17,19]
- Mowing TE+ TFG/ergotized seed heads and curing hay reduces concentrations; unlikely to eliminate completely
  - Do *not* mow TE+ TFG pastures less than 3 inches (7.5 cm); the bottom 2 inches (5 cm) potentially contain high ergovaline concentrations.
- Replace TE+ TFG pastures
  - Other grasses/nontoxic/less toxic novel E+ fescue varieties

- ○ TE+ TFG may eventually contaminate novel E+ pastures
  - ■ Endophyte-free tall fescue not hardy/persistent enough to succeed in these areas
- ○ Novel E+ tall fescue still susceptible to *C purpurea* (see **Fig. 3**)
  - ■ Monitor for ergot

Other resources

- Additional information on "fescue toxicosis" and various approaches to mitigating effects of EAs on livestock, especially pasture management and renovation[1–4,15,17]
  - ○ Extension and research publications by agronomy, animal science, and veterinary experts at North Carolina State University, the University of Georgia, the University of Kentucky, the University of Missouri, and other universities in the "fescue belt"

DISCLOSURE

No disclosure.

FUNDING

USDA/ARS 58-6227-8-041, Managed reductions of problems associated with fescue toxicosis at both plant and animal levels. **Co-Principal Investigator**, USDA-ARS Missouri-Arkansas Fescue Endophyte Cooperative Agreement (≈ $200,000/year), 2003-2010 (Annual Renewal). Effects of perphenazine and reserpine on pony mares with prolonged gestation. **Co-Principal Investigator**, USDA Formula Funds ($15,000), 1994-1995.

REFERENCES

1. Evans TJ, Rottinghaus GE, Casteel SW, et al. Fescue. In: Plumlee K, editor. Clinical veterinary toxicology. St Louis (MO): Mosby; 2004. p. 243–50.
2. Roberts C. Tall fescue toxicosis. MU Guide G 4669, MU Extension, University of Missouri-Columbia, 2000, Available at: https://extension.missouri.edu/publications/g46692000, Accessed October 1, 2023.
3. Smith SR, et al. Tall fescue toxicity for horses: literature review and Kentucky's successful pasture evaluation program. Proc Fescue Toxicosis SRM/AFGC Annual Meeting, January 26 - January 31, 2008 in Louisville, KY.
4. Phipps K, et al: Comparison of commercially available novel-endophyte tall fescue forage varieties. AG-910, NC State Extension, 2021, Available at: https://content.ces.ncsu.edu/comparison-of-commercially-available-novel-endophyte-tall-fescue-forage-varieties, Accessed October 1, 2023.
5. Burrows GE, Tyrl RJ. Toxic plants of North America. 2nd edition. Ames (IA): John Wiley and sons; 2013. p. 940–9.
6. Young CA, Schardl CL, Panaccione DG, et al. Genetics, genomics and evolution of ergot alkaloid diversity. Toxins (Basel) 2015;7(4):1273–302.
7. Florea S, Panaccione DG, Schardl CL. Ergot Alkaloids of the family Clavicipitaceae. Phytopathology 2017;107(5):504–18.
8. Kerr LA, Kelch WJ, in Howard JL, et al. Current veterinary therapy 4: Food animal practice. Philadelphia: Saunders; 1999. p. 263–4.
9. Hill NS, Thompson FN, Stuedemann JA, et al. Ergot alkaloid transport across ruminant gastric tissues. J Anim Sci 2001;79:542–9.

10. Evans TJ, Rottinghaus GE, Casteel SW, et al. Ergot. In: Plumlee K, editor. Clinical veterinary toxicology. St Louis (MO): Mosby; 2004. p. 239–43.
11. Evans TJ. The endocrine disruptive effects of ergopeptine alkaloids on pregnant mares. Vet Clin North Am Equine Pract 2011;27(1):165–73.
12. Ireland FA, Loch WE, Worthy K, et al. Effects of bromocriptine and perphenazine on prolactin and progesterone concentrations in pregnant pony mares during late gestation. J Reprod Fertil 1991;92:179–86.
13. Evans TJ, Youngquist RS, Loch WE, et al. A comparison of the relative efficacies of domperidone and reserpine in treating equine "fescue toxicosis". Proc Am Assoc Equine Pract 1999;45:207–9.
14. Evans TJ. The effects of bromocriptine, domperidone, and reserpine on circulating, maternal levels of progestins, estrogens, and prolactin in pregnant pony mares. Columbia, MO: Master's Thesis, University of Missouri-Columbia; 1996.
15. Evans TJ. Fescue toxicosis. In: Hovda LR, Benson D, Poppenga RH, et al, editors. Equine toxicology (5-minute consult). Hoboken, NJ: Wiley-Blackwell; 2022. p. 220–5.
16. Strickland JR, Looper ML, Matthews JC, et al. Board-invited review: St. Anthony's Fire in livestock: causes, mechanisms, and potential solutions. J Anim Sci 2011; 89:1603–26.
17. Kenyon SL, Roberts CA, Kallenbach RL, et al. Vertical distribution of ergot alkaloids in the vegetative canopy of tall fescue. Crop Science 2018;58(2):925–31.
18. Gupta RC, Evans TJ, Nicholson SS. Ergot and Fescue Toxicoses. In: Gupta RC, editor. Veterinary Toxicology: Basic and clinical Principles. 3rd edition. New York: Academic Press/Elsevier, Inc.; 2018. p. 995–1001.
19. Cross DL, Redmond LM, Strickland JR. Equine fescue toxicosis: signs and solutions. J Anim Sci 1995;73:899–908.
20. McDowell KJ, Moore ES, Parks AG, et al. Vasoconstriction in horses caused by endophyte-infected tall fescue seed is detected with Doppler ultrasonography. J Anim Sci 2013;91(4):1677–84.
21. Klotz JL, McDowell KJ. Tall fescue ergot alkaloids are vasoactive in equine vasculature. J Anim Sci 2017;95(11):5151–60.
22. Vivrette S, Stebbins ME, Martin O, et al. Cardiorespiratory and thermoregulatory effects of endophyte-infected fescue in exercising horses. Journal of Equine Veterinary Science 2001;21(2):65–7.
23. Webb GW, Ford JA, Webb SP, et al. Effect of Ergovaline Ingestion on Recovery of Horses Subjected to an Anaerobic Standard Exercise Test. Journal of Equine Veterinary Science 2010;30(12):705–10.
24. Rohrbach BW, Green EM, Oliver JW, et al. Aggregate risk study of *exposure* to endophyte-infected (*Acremonium coenophialum*) tall fescue as a risk factor for laminitis in horses. Am J Vet Res 1995;56:22–6.
25. Bennett-Wimbush K, Loch WE, Plata-Madrid H, et al. The effects of perphenazine and bromocriptine on follicular dynamics and endocrine profiles in anestrous pony mares. Theriogenology 1998;49:717–33.
26. Looper ML, Rorie RW, Person CN, et al. Influence of toxic endophyte-infected fescue on sperm characteristics and endocrine factors of yearling Brahman-influenced bulls. J Anim Sci 2008;87(3):1184–91.
27. Burke JM, Spiers DE, Kojima FN, et al. Interaction of endophyte-infected fescue and heat stress on ovarian function in the beef heifer. Biol Reprod 2001;65:260–8.
28. Fayrer-Hosken R, Stanley A, Hill N, et al. Effect of feeding fescue seed containing ergot alkaloid toxins on stallion spermatogenesis and sperm cells. Reprod Domest Anim 2012;47(6):1017–26.

29. Stuedemann JA, Hill NS, Thompson FN, et al. Urinary and biliary excretion of ergot alkaloids from steers that grazed endophyte-infected tall fescue. J Anim Sci 1998;76:2146–54.
30. Crews C. Analysis of ergot alkaloids. Toxins (Basel) 2015;7(6):2024–50.
31. Krska R, Crews C. Significance, chemistry and determination of ergot alkaloids: a review. Food Addit Contam Part A Chem Anal Control Expo Risk Assess 2008; 25(6):722–31.
32. Rudolph W, Remane D, Wissenbach DK, et al. Development and validation of an ultrahigh performance liquid chromatography-high resolution tandem mass spectrometry assay for nine toxic alkaloids from endophyte-infected pasture grasses in horse serum. J Chromatogr A 2018;1560:35–44.
33. Cherewyk JE, Parker SE, Blakley BR, et al. Assessment of the vasoactive effects of the (S)-epimers of ergot alkaloids in vitro. J Anim Sci 2020;98(7). https://doi. org/10.1093/jas/skaa203. Corrigendum in J Anim Sci 99(4): skab103. doi: 10.1093/jas/skab103, 2021.
34. Rottinghaus GE, Garner GB, Cornell CN, et al. HPLC method for quantitating ergovaline in endophyte-infested tall fescue: seasonal variation of ergovaline levels in stems with leaf sheaths, leaf blades, and seed heads. J. Agric. Food Chem. 1991;39(1):112–5.
35. Rottinghaus GE, Schultz LM, Ross PF, et al. An HPLC method for the detection of ergot in ground and pelleted feeds. J Vet Diagn Invest 1993;5(2):242–7.
36. Kallenbach RL, BILL E. BILL E. KUNKLE INTERDISCIPLINARY BEEF SYMPOSIUM: Coping with tall fescue toxicosis: Solutions and realities. J Anim Sci 2015;93:5487–95.
37. Alfaro GF, Moisá SJ. Fescue toxicosis: a detrimental condition that requires a multiapproach solution. Anim Front 2022;12(5):23–8.
38. Lucas KM, Koltes DA, Meyer LR, et al. Identification of breed differences in known and new fescue toxicosis associated phenotypes in charolais-and hereford-sired crossbred beef cows. Animals (Basel) 2021;11(10):2830.
39. Britt JL, Greene MA, Bridges WC, et al. Ergot alkaloid exposure during gestation alters. I. Maternal characteristics and placental development of pregnant ewes1. J Anim Sci 2019;97(4):1874–90.
40. Greene MA, Britt JL, Bertrand JK, et al. Feeding tall fescue seed during mid and late gestation influences subsequent postnatal growth, puberty, and carcass quality of offspring. Animals (Basel) 2020;10(10):1859.
41. Bourke CA, Hunt E, Watson R. Fescue-associated oedema of horses grazing on endophyte-inoculated tall fescue grass (Festuca arundinacea) pastures. Aust Vet J 2009;87(12):492–8.
42. Finch SC, Munday JS, Sutherland BL, et al. Further investigation of equine fescue oedema induced by Mediterranean tall fescue (Lolium arundinaceum) infected with selected fungal endophytes (Epichloë coenophiala). N Z Vet J 2017;65(6):322–6.
43. Dierking RM, Kallenbach RL. Mediterranean and Continental Tall Fescue: II. Effects of Cold, Nonfreezing Temperatures on Leaf Extension, Proline, Fructan, and Abscisic Acid. Crop Science 2012;52(1):460–9.
44. Munday JS, Finch SC, Vlaming JB, et al. Pathological changes seen in horses in New Zealand grazing Mediterranean tall fescue (Lolium arundinaceum) infected with selected endophytes (Epichloë coenophiala) causing equine fescue oedema. N Z Vet J 2017;65(3):147–51.
45. Dechra Veterinary Products: Package insert for EQUIDONE® Gel. Revised 8/ 2023. Available at: https://dailymed.nlm.nih.gov/dailymed/fda/fdaDrugXsl.cfm? setid=e55d075e-2fe2-4405-b57a-59b85067e0c0&type=display.

Cantharidin

Karyn Bischoff, DVM, MS, MPH

KEYWORDS

- Cantharidin • Blister beetles • Hypocalcemia • Colic • Hypomagnesemia • Ulcers
- Myocardial necrosis

KEY POINTS

- Blister beetle poisoning is reported over much of North America and, in horses, is almost exclusively linked to feeding alfalfa.
- The toxic principle, cantharidin, is a blistering agent that acts by inhibiting the protein phosphatase 2A on the cell membrane, causing acantholysis of epithelium, leading to blistering and subsequent erosions and ulcerations.
- Cantharidin can cause myocardial necrosis, and elevated cardiac troponin 1 is frequently reported in affected horses.
- Along with colic, hypocalcemia and hypomagnesemia are most frequently reported in affected horses.
- Ending exposure and aggressive treatment with decontamination, pain control, gastroprotective agents, and correction of dehydration and electrolyte abnormalities are critical for patient survival.

INTRODUCTION

Cantharidin toxicosis, or blister beetle poisoning, has been reported in horses over much of the United States, northern Mexico, and Canada and is almost exclusively associated with feeding alfalfa hay.[1–6] Though poisonings have been seen as far east as New York, they are most common in the Midwestern and Southwestern United States, particularly in Texas and Oklahoma.[3,7] Sale and movement of alfalfa hay and hay products across North America broadens the potential range of cantharidin toxicosis. The disease is caused by ingestion of blister beetles, which are of the genus *Epicauta*, that have become incorporated into alfalfa hay during harvest and crimping.[5,6] Mature blister beetles are attracted to alfalfa flowers, upon which they feed, and are thus likely to occur in hay that was harvested in bloom.[4] Blister beetles are toxic to horses because they contain the double-ringed diterpenoid compound cantharidin, a colorless, odorous agent with vesicant actions.[8–10]

There are thousands of species of blister beetle, and hundreds of species reported in the United States, though not all have been associated with poisoning.[8,9] The most common species associated with blister beetle poisonings include the following:[3,7]

Department of Population Medicine and Diagnostic Sciences, Cornell University College of Veterinary Medicine, New York State Animal Health Diagnostic Center, PO Box 5786, Ithaca, NY 14853, USA
E-mail address: KLB72@cornell.edu

Vet Clin Equine 40 (2024) 113–119
https://doi.org/10.1016/j.cveq.2023.08.002
0749-0739/24/Published by Elsevier Inc.

- *Epicauta occidentalis* and *E texexa*, three-striped blister beetles
- *E comferta* and *E pennsylvanica*, black blister beetles
- *E paradalis*, spotted blister beetles
- *E albida*, green blister beetles.

The male blister beetle produces cantharidin as a defensive chemical, and it is transferred to the female as a nuptial gift to protect her eggs.[6,9,11]

Historical medical uses of cantharidin isolated from blister beetles include wart removal and as a veterinary vesicant or blistering agent.[12,13]

DISCUSSION
Toxicity

- Blister beetles can contain more than 12%, dry matter, cantharidin, which is toxic to horses at a dose of less than 1 mg/kg body weight.[2,6,8]
- Cantharidin is rapidly absorbed through the gastrointestinal tract and rapidly excreted via the urinary tract.[2,6]
- Cantharidin binds to and inhibits a specific membrane protein, protein phosphatase type 2A (PP2A), which acts on serine/threonine.[1]
- Cantharidin also inhibits PP1.[8]
- The major action of cantharidin is to produce epithelial acantholysis, resulting in blisters progressing to erosions and ulcers.[8]
- Cantharidin also prevents activation of transcription factors involved in activation of osteoclasts, which may contribute to the hypocalcemia reported in blister beetle toxicosis.[8,14]
- Inhibition of parathyroid hormone secretion has also been proposed as a cause of hypocalcemia, and may be related to inhibition of PP1 or to hypomagnesemia.[14]

Clinical signs: Although primarily considered an equine problem, cantharidin toxicosis has been reported in other species including alpacas, sheep, and emu.[2,8,10] Clinical signs of poisoning are dose dependent and general have a rapid, abrupt onset, though onset can be delayed up to 2 days.[5,6,8] The most common clinical signs refer to abdominal pain and can include the following:

- Signs of colic such as restlessness, irritability, sweating, pawing at the ground, grunting, trembling, clenched teeth, and reluctance to move.[4–6,8]
- Anorexia or feed refusal.[6,15]
- Signs of oral irritation can include submerging of the muzzle in water with or without polydipsia, and ptyalism.[4,6,8,15]
- Tachycardia.[4,5,8,15]
- Mucous membranes can be hyperemic or dark, and capillary refill time is often diminished.[4,6,8]
- Tachypnea is often seen, and synchronous diaphragmatic flutter has been occasionally reported.[6,8,15]
- Elevated body temperature early in the clinical course.[6,15]
- Dehydration[6]
- Dysuria, which may include polyuria, pollakiuria, and sometimes microscopic or gross hematuria.[5,6,8]
- Signs of central nervous system involvement, including depression, head pressing, and disorientation, have been reported, sometimes in the absence of gastrointestinal distress.[5]
- Terminal seizures are frequently seen.[5]
- Some horses die before clinical signs are observed.[5,6]

- Secondary laminitis is common in horses recovering from cantharidin toxicosis.[16]

Clinical pathology findings often include the following:

- Hemoconcentration.[6,8]
- Hypocalcemia within the first 6 hours post-exposure, persisting for more than 48 hours in the absence of treatment.[6,15] Hypocalcemia is one of the most common clinical findings, and was reported in 9 out of the 10 affected horses in one study and 75% of the horses in another.[5,8]
- Hypomagnesemia is also an early finding and can be protracted, but was only reported in 2/10 horses in one study.[5,6,15]
- Hypokalemia has been reported early in the clinical course and tends to be transient and mild.[6,15]
- Hyperglycemia is commonly reported.[6,8]
- Though urinary tract involvement is commonly reported, azotemia was only seen in 3 of the 10 horses in one study.[5]
- Elevated creatine kinase has been associated with a poor prognosis.[6,15]
- Elevated cardiac troponin 1 was seen in about half of clinical cases.[8]

Postmortem Lesions

Many of the postmortem lesions are due to the acantholytic effects of cantharidin on epithelium, particularly in the gastrointestinal and urinary tracts.

- Gross postmortem lesions are frequently seen, but may be absent, particularly after a peracute clinical course.[5]
- A study found that 14 of the 24 necropsied horses had mucosal erythema in the gastrointestinal tract, including the gastric and intestinal mucosa, and a few had erosions and ulcerations affecting the oral cavity, esophagus, or stomach.[5]
- Mucosal necrosis and swelling were associated with the glandular mucosa of the stomach.[6]
- Intestinal contents are frequently reported to be watery.[6,15]
- Mucosal vesicles or hemorrhage and can affect the urinary bladder, ureters, and renal pelvis.[5,6]
- Renal tubular necrosis has also been noted.[6] Myocardial lesions were reported in 1 out of the 24 necropsied horses in one study.[5]
- Lesions are associated with myocardial necrosis and depend on dose and duration of exposure, heart lesions were not seen in horses that died within 2 days of exposure.[6,15,17]

Diagnosis

A tentative diagnosis of cantharidin toxicosis can be made based on the combination of clinical signs, clinical pathology findings, particularly hypocalcemia, and the presence of alfalfa in the diet. Blister beetle poisoning can be distinguished from other causes of colic by the hypocalcemia and hypomagnesemia that are most consistently associated with cantharidin.[5,6]

Detection of blister beetles in the feed or, rarely, stomach contents, supports the diagnosis (**Fig. 1**). Definitive diagnosis requires detection of cantharidin using gas chromatography with mass spectrometry or liquid chromatography.[2,6,8] The samples of choice are stomach contents and urine, but false negatives are possible if samples are not collected soon after exposure.[2,6,8] Urine is negative for cantharidin within 3 to 4 days of exposure, and intravenous fluid therapy can dilute the urinary concentration of cantharidin below the detection limit of analytical methods used for cantharidin

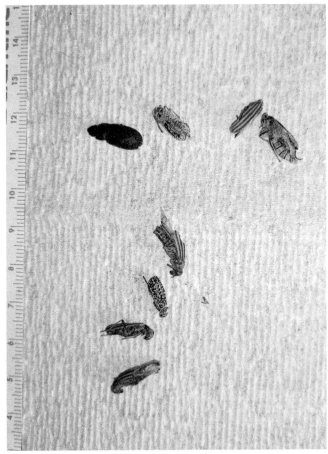

Fig. 1. Crushed and fragmented blister beetles (*Epicauta* spp.) of various species, and other insects, recovered from a flake of alfalfa hay.

detection.[6] Cantharidin has been detected in the kidney, cecal contents, and feed from affected animals.[3] Cantharidin concentrations in the liver are unlikely to be detectable.[2]

Treatment

Treatment for cantharidin toxicosis is predominantly supportive care and involves the following:

- Elimination of exposure
  - Ending exposure involves changing the feed source by eliminating the alfalfa source of blister beetles from the diet.[6,8]
- Decreasing absorption of ingested cantharidin
  - Administration of activated charcoal by nasogastric tube at a dose of 1 to 3 g/kg body weight has been recommended to decrease cantharidin absorption.[8,16]
    - Activated charcoal (without a cathartic) can be administered every 12 hours up to 3 times.[16]

- Pain management
  - Because of the ulcerative nature of blister beetle toxicosis, use of corticosteroids and nonsteroidal anti-inflammatory drugs may be ill advised.[8]
    - α-2 agonists
      - Xylazine 0.3 to 0.5 mg/kg IV has been used for short-term analgesia.[16]
      - Alternately, detomidine 0.01 to 0.02 mg/kg IV has been used for short-term analgesia.[16]
    - Opioids
      - Butorphanol has been used for pain control in horses and alpacas because the κ-opioid receptor agonist effect may provide more pain control than μ-receptor agonists in cantharidin toxicosis.[8,16]
- Loading dose of 20 μg/kg IV in horses.[16]
- Constant rate infusion of 13 μg/kg/hour diluted in lactated Ringer's solution.[16]
- Gastroprotectants
  - Gastroprotectants, such as sucralfate and omeprazole, are critical due to mucosal damage and will also help to moderate discomfort.[18]
- Fluid and electrolyte support.
  - Fluid therapy is used as needed based on blood work to treat calcium and magnesium deficits and hemoconcentration and to provide renal support.

Oral mineral oil was historically used to treat blister beetle ingestion in horses and other species, but has fallen out of favor; experimental rodents treated with mineral oil after oral dosing with cantharidin had poorer outcomes and there was evidence that the mineral oil increased cantharidin absorption from the gastrointestinal tract.[19]

Prognosis is considered poor.[6] One study found that 51% of the affected horses survived after aggressive treatment.[5,6] Horses alive 2 days after onset are likely to survive, but treatment may be protracted for 14 days.[5,6] Elevated creatine kinase and persistent tachycardia and tachypnea are considered poor prognostic indicators.[6,15]

Prevention: Due to the severe impact on animal health and welfare, and the protracted course of aggressive therapy required to treat blister beetle poisoning, preventing exposure to cantharidin in horses and other animals is of critical importance. Historically, blister beetles were associated with alfalfa hay cuttings that took place in or after June in the southern United States and after August in the central Midwestern states, and early cuttings before bloom may be less likely to be contaminated.[4,6] Inspection of alfalfa fields for beetle swarms before cutting and crimping could be helpful.[6] Because they swarm, beetles may be concentrated in a bale or a few flakes of alfalfa hay, thus inspection of individual flakes for beetles is warranted, but time consuming and potentially impractical, and beetles can still be missed.[6,8] Alfalfa cubes, wafers, and pellets can also be contaminated.[8] The dilution factor in pellets makes them less likely to contain enough cantharidin to be problematic, though contamination of alfalfa pellets has been reported.[3,8] Storage does not diminish the toxicity of cantharidin.[6]

SUMMARY

The biological effects of cantharidin, the toxic component of blister beetle species in the *Epicauta* genus, have long been known to medicine.[12,13] Cantharidin, which is eliminated in the urine, is a potent vesicant which acts on a specific membrane protein, PP2A, to cause acantholysis in epithelium, resulting in blisters, erosions, and ulcerations, and can affect the gastrointestinal and urinary tracts of horses that ingest blister beetles.[1,2] Blister beetles tend to swarm in alfalfa fields that are in bloom, and if alfalfa is harvested and crimped while swarms are present, alfalfa products (hay, cubes, pellets) become contaminated with cantharidin.[3] Though cantharidin toxicosis is most common in the Midwest, in particular in Texas and Oklahoma, blister beetles are found across much of North America, and alfalfa products may be shipped to locations distant from where they were produced.[3,4]

Clinical signs of cantharidin toxicosis are dose dependent, but the painful mucosal ulceration associated with blister beetle ingestion can cause colic and dysuria.[5] The combined history and clinical findings of alfalfa feeding, evidence of colic, hypocalcemia, and hypomagnesemia are highly suggestive of blister beetle toxicosis.[4,5] Myocardial damage can occur, leading to increased creatine kinase and cardiac troponin 1 concentrations in the serum. Blister beetles may be evident in the hay, supporting the diagnosis, but definitive diagnosis requires analysis of urine or gastric contents for cantharidin.[2]

Treatment of affected horses is primarily symptomatic and supportive and relies on ending exposure, decreasing absorption with activated charcoal, pain control, use of gastroprotectants, and fluid and electrolyte replacement.[6] About half of horses with severe cantharidin toxicosis are expected to survive with aggressive therapy, thus prevention through careful selection of uncontaminated alfalfa is warranted.[5]

CLINICS CARE POINTS

- Eliminate the source of exposure by removing contaminated food.[6,8]
- Decrease absorption of ingested cantharidin by administering activated charcoal.[8,16]
  - Activated charcoal (without a cathartic) can be administered every 12 hours up to 3 times.[16]
- Pain management with butorphanol has been successful.[8,16]
  - Loading dose of 20 μg/kg IV in horses.[16]
  - Constant rate infusion of 13 μg/kg/hr diluted in lactated Ringer's solution.[16]
- Gastroprotectants, such as sucralfate and omeprazole, are critical and will also help to moderate discomfort.[18]
- Fluid and electrolyte support are required to treat dehydration, hypocalcemia, and hypomagnesemia.

DISCLOSURE

The authors has nothing to disclose.

REFERENCES

1. Li YM, Casida JE. Cantharidin-binding protein: identification as protein phosphatase 2A. Proc Natl Acad Sci USA 1992;89:11867–70.
2. Ray AC, Post LO, Hurst JM, et al. Evaluation of an analytical method for the diagnosis of cantharidin toxicosis due to ingestion of blister beetles (Epicauta lemniscata) by horses and sheep. Am J Vet Res 1980;41:932–3.
3. Edwards WC, Edwards RM, Ogden L, et al. Cantharidin content of two species of Oklahoma blister beetles associated with toxicosis in horses. Vet Hum Toxicol 1989;31:442–4.
4. Beasley VR, Wolf GA, Fischer DC, et al. Cantharidin toxicosis in horses. J Am Vet Med Assoc 1983;182:283–4.
5. Helman RG, Edwards WC. Clinical features of blister beetle poisoning in equids: 70 cases (1983-1996). J Am Vet Med Assoc 1997;211:1018–21.

6. Schmitz DG. Cantharidin Toxicosis in Horses. J Vet Intern Med 1989;3:208–15.
7. Ray AC, Kyle AL, Murphy MJ, et al. Etiologic agents, incidence, and improved diagnostic methods of cantharidin toxicosis in horses. Am J Vet Res 1989;50:187–91.
8. Simpson KM, Streeter RN, De Souza P, et al. Cantharidin toxicosis in 2 alpacas. Can Vet J 2013;54:456–62.
9. Falck B. Spanish Fly—Cantharidin's Alter Ego. JAMA Dermatology 2018;154:51.
10. Barr AC, Wigle WL, Flory W, et al. Cantharidin Poisoning of Emu Chicks by Ingestion of Pyrota Insulata. J Vet Diagn Invest 1998;10:77–9.
11. Carrel JE, Eisner T. Cantharidin: Potent Feeding Deterrent to Insects. Science 1974;183:755–7.
12. Appelgren L-E. Spanish flies in the veterinary pharmacy in Skara–their medicinal use yesterday and to day. Hist Med Vet 2010;35:35–48.
13. Cumming MS. Blisters, beetles, and beliefs. Vet Herit 1995;18:3–10.
14. Kim MH, Shim KS, Kim SH. Inhibitory effect of cantharidin on osteoclast differentiation and bone resorption. Arch Pharm Res (Seoul) 2010;33:457–62.
15. Shawley RV, Rolf LL. Experimental cantharidiasis in the horse. Am J Vet Res 1984;45:2261–6.
16. Holbrook TC. Treating cantharidin toxicosis. Comp Equine 2009;4:353–7.
17. Zhang Y, Yu Y, Zhang J, et al. Biomarkers of myocardial injury in rats after cantharidin poisoning: Application for postmortem diagnosis and estimation of postmortem interval. Sci Rep 2020;10:12069.
18. Bishop RC, Kemper AM, Wilkins PA, et al. Effect of omeprazole and sucralfate on gastrointestinal injury in a fasting/NSAID model. Equine Vet J 2022;54:829–37.
19. Qualls HJ, Holbrook TC, Gilliam LL, et al. Evaluation of Efficacy of Mineral Oil, Charcoal, and Smectite in a Rat Model of Equine Cantharidin Toxicosis. J Vet Intern Med 2013;27:1179–84.

Blue Green Algae

Scott A. Fritz, DVM[a],*, Savannah Charnas, DVM, MPH[b],
Steve Ensley, DVM, PhD[a]

KEYWORDS

- Blue green algae • Harmful algal blooms • Cyanotoxin • Equine • Horse

KEY POINTS

- There are several fresh water cyanotoxins produced by blue green algae that can potentially affect equines.
- While equine-specific blue green algae toxicosis is not commonly reported, expected clinical signs are related to hepatotoxicity and neurotoxicity.
- Treatment is largely symptomatic, and the prognosis is grave for animals that develop clinical signs.
- Preventing exposure via management practices is essential.

INTRODUCTION

Harmful algal blooms (HAB) have become increasingly common due to warming climates, over enrichment of nutrients such as nitrogen and phosphorus (eutrophication), and increased industrial and agricultural practices.[1,2] They are defined as dense growths of algae or cyanobacteria that lower dissolved water oxygen levels and produce toxins that harm animal life.[3] In relation to equines, HABs are commonly found in water sources such as farm ponds or dugouts, and are usually due to warm water temperatures, phosphorus or nitrogen- rich fertilizer contamination, and/or excrement runoff.[4] Examples of cyanobacterial blooms can be seen in **Figs. 1** and **2**. Note the variation in color of the different blooms. These bloom-forming algal species have the ability to produce cyano-toxins or phyco-toxins, which are secondary metabolites capable of causing damage to organisms on a cellular level.[5] While phycotoxin poisoning is seen in both salt and fresh water bodies, freshwater phycotoxicoses are more applicable to equines and have been reported in mammals, wild and domestic birds, and aquatic invertebrates, either through direct ingestion of contaminated water or indirectly through biomagnification.[3] Future research is needed to better elucidate these toxicoses, and to obtain more specific data relating to toxicity in horses.

[a] Department of Anatomy and Physiology, Kansas State University College of Veterinary Medicine, 1620 Denison Avenue, 228 Coles Hall, Manhattan, KS 66506, USA; [b] Kansas State Veterinary Diagnostic Laboratory, 1800 Denison Avenue, Manhattan, KS 66506, USA
* Corresponding author.
E-mail address: scottfritz@vet.k-state.edu

Vet Clin Equine 40 (2024) 121–132
https://doi.org/10.1016/j.cveq.2023.10.006
vetequine.theclinics.com

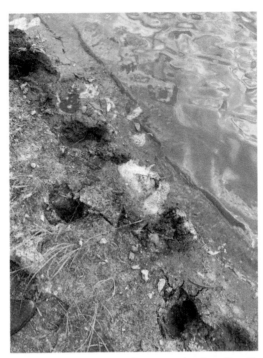

Fig. 1. Blue-green algae can be seen in a hoof print on the shoreline. (*Image courtesy*: Scott Fritz.)

FRESHWATER TOXINS
Cylindrospermopsin

Cylindrospermopsin (CYN) is an alkaloid cytotoxin that is highly water soluble and environmentally stable. As such, it is more likely to be suspended in water, making it harder to filter as a possible treatment.[3] CYN-producing species are widely distributed in areas that include the Midwestern United States, though are commonly found in subtropical to temperate climate zones.[3,6] No significant color change is appreciated with their presence, so they are difficult to visually identify in possibly contaminated water.[6] The first species noted to produce CYN was *Raphidiopsis raciborskii*, and most CYN-producing algae can similarly be found from the orders of Nostocales or Oscillatoriales.[6] Specific species include *Chrysoporum ovalisporum*, *Umezakia natans*, *Aphanizomenon flos-aquae*, *Aph. gracile*, *Raphidiopsis mediterranea*, *Raphidiopsis curvata*, *Anabaena bergii*, *Lyngbya wollei*, *Ana. lapponica*, *Phormidium ambiguum*, *Oscillatoria* sp., *Ana. affinis*, *Raphidiopsis catemaco*, *Raphidiopsis phillippinensis*, and *Planktothrix agardhii*.[6]

CYNs are primarily hepatotoxic but do have the ability to affect other organs such as lungs, kidneys, stomach, thymus, spleen, and small intestine. Additionally, they are cytotoxic, genotoxic, immunotoxic, neurotoxic, and potentially carcinogenic due to their primary mechanism of action being the inhibition of protein synthesis.[5,6] Currently, there are no known case reports in equines, though the first livestock mortality case can be traced back to Queensland, AUS in 1997. Three cows and ten calves died from contaminated water, and lesions included pale livers, liver fibrosis, liver necrosis, edema, and both epicardial and intestinal hemorrhages.[6] Currently, there is no

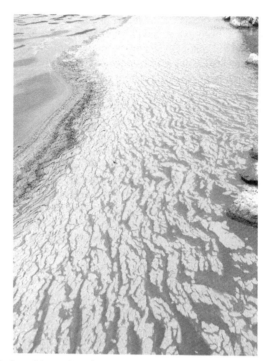

Fig. 2. A harmful algae bloom (HAB) concentrating on the shoreline after being blown by prevailing winds. Significant exposures can occur when animals drink from the affected areas. (*Image courtesy:* Scott Fritz.)

established LD_{50} dose for horses, but experimental LD_{50} doses in mice via intraperitoneal (IP) injection were found to be 2.1 mg/kg over 24 hours, and 0.2 mg/kg over 5 to 6 days. Inflammation, swelling, fat accumulation, and increased hepatocellular vacuolation and necrosis were observed in the livers of exposed mice.[6] Kidney lesions included interstitial nephritis, decreased glomerular erythrocytes, epithelial cell necrosis, and glycogen and protein deposition in the renal tubules. Both the kidney and liver had noted radioactivity, and bloodwork revealed elevations in alanine transaminase (ALT), sorbitol dehydrogenase (SDH), and blood urea nitrogen (BUN), while protein concentration was reduced.[6]

Microcystins and Nodularins

Microcystin (MC) is a cyanotoxin with a cyclic peptide structure that allows it to be extremely resistant to degradation.[7] There are currently over 275 congeners with the most common being MC-LR, MC-YR, and MC-RR.[8] MCs are a well-known hazard to livestock, fisheries, wildlife, and human health due to their increasing presence, though there are few case reports specifically involving horses.[9] Nodularin (ND) is a cyanotoxin with a similar structure, though it is a cyclic pentapeptide.[10] There are ten naturally occurring isoforms of NDs, though NOD-R is the isoform most commonly seen in HABs.[10] They are mainly produced by *Nodularia spumigena* while the other most common strain is *Nodularia sphaerocarpa*.[10] Both MCs and NDs share the same mechanism of action, which is to bind and inhibit serine and threonine protein phosphatases.[3] Ultimately this causes excess phosphorylation of essential proteins leading to oxidative injury, collapse of cytoskeletal structures, inhibition of gluconeogenesis, enhanced glycolysis, necrosis, and apoptosis.[3] The liver is affected similarly by both MCs and NDs via hepatocytes uptaking both cyanotoxins via organic anion transport polypeptides (OATPs, or bile acid transporters). OATPs are most concentrated in hepatocytes making them more susceptible to uptake and subsequent damage.[9] Since OATPs are widespread in other organ systems, they can affect both the GI tract and the kidneys in a similar fashion.[3,9]

While there are no specific LD_{50} doses established for horses, laboratory experiments with mice have provided a range of doses. For MCs, LD_{50} doses range from 50 μg/kg to 11 mg/kg depending on the congener, species, and route. The oral LD_{50} in mice was found to be 10.9 mg/kg for MC-LR, and the IP LD_{50} in mice for MC-LR was 50 μg/kg.[7] For NDs, the LD_{50} via IP injection in mice ranged from 50 μg/kg to 150 μg/kg.[10] Most animals that are exposed die within a few hours, and the most common route of exposure is either direct ingestion from water, or ingestion through grooming algal mats off their coat.[7] Clinical signs include diarrhea, vomiting, pale mucous membranes, weakness, and shock. Those that do not immediately die can shows signs of hypoglycemia, hyperkalemia, recumbency, nervousness, and convulsions. Additionally, animals that survive acute toxicosis have the possibility to display hepatic photosensitization. It is also worth noting that the carcinogenic effects of both MCs and NDs have been documented in humans, with primary liver and colorectal cancer developing after prolonged exposure.[7]

Anatoxin-a and Saxitoxin

Both anatoxin-a and saxitoxin are neurotoxic alkaloids that have been responsible for acute blue-green algae toxicosis in animals throughout the globe due to their widespread distribution.[11] While it is more common to see saxitoxins in bodies of salt water, there are currently 41 and 15 freshwater variants of anatoxin-a and saxitoxin-producing blue-green algae species, respectively. Examples of anatoxin-a-producing species include *Anabaena circinalis, Anabaena flos-aquae, Aphanizomenon gracile,* and *Oscillatoria agardhii,* while species such as *Aphanizomenon favaloroi, L wollei, Phormidium,* and *Woronichinia* are some of the known saxitoxin producers.[11] Anatoxin-a and saxitoxins are water soluble, and both are pH and temperature dependent. Saxitoxins are most stable in a pH range of 2 to 4, and begin to degrade the more alkaline the water becomes.[11] Additionally, they are most stable at temperatures closer to 68°F, and when they do degrade they become up to 6 × more toxic as they are converted into more potent dicarbamoyl-gonyautoxins that can last for as long as 10 days. Similar to saxitoxins, anatoxin-a persists more in water with temperatures below 68°F, pHs less than 3, and with less sunlight. Unlike saxitoxins, however, anatoxin-a will degrade into non-toxic forms. There is the possibility that both neurotoxins can accumulate in terrestrial plants via absorption from the soil, though all proven instances have been seen under experimental conditions only.[11]

The method of action for anatoxin-a is to mimic acetylcholine and bind to acetylcholine receptors. As they cannot be degraded by acetylcholinesterase, muscles become overstimulated leading to fatigue and possibly respiratory failure if the exposure is severe enough.[11] Saxitoxins operate by blocking sodium channels and affecting nerve conduction, and this also can result in respiratory paralysis if muscle stimulation is decreased sufficiently. While its salt water variant (paralytic shellfish toxin) is known to be extremely toxic, the freshwater form is less so as it contains a hydrophobic side chain that causes a decrease in sodium channel receptor binding.[11] Like the other toxins, there is not an established toxic dose for horses, though experimental studies have been performed in mice. The LD_{50} via IP injection for anatoxin-a was found to be 200 to 250 μg/kg, and 5.5 to 10 μg/kg for saxitoxins.[11] The oral exposure LD_{50} for both neurotoxins is higher at greater than 5000 µg/kg for anatoxin-a in mice, and 7 to 15 µg/ kg in humans.[11] General clinical signs seen are related to both the neurologic and respiratory systems, though visual disturbances, GI upset, and dermatologic symptoms are also common. Specifically, in anatoxin-a acute effects are convulsions, muscle twitching, paralysis, and respiratory failure, with deaths being reported within minutes to hours postexposure. The acute effects of saxitoxin exposure are similar to their salt water varieties where symptoms include vomiting, diarrhea, excessive sweating, salivation, and headache. Unlike their saltwater counterparts, there are no confirmed deaths from freshwater saxitoxin exposure.[11]

Guanitoxin

Formerly known as anatoxin-a(s), guanitoxins (GNTs) are a naturally occurring organophosphate that is primarily produced by species of the genera *Dolichospermum* and *Sphaerospermopsis*.[11,12] While they are less common than other cyanotoxins, significant amounts of GNT have been detected throughout various bodies of water in North America, South America, Europe, and Asia.[12,13] GNTs are less stable at higher water temperatures and in water that is slightly alkaline, though the exact half-life is undetermined.[12] Most animal exposures are due to oral ingestion of contaminated water sources, and GNT has demonstrated bioavailability in both the stomach and intestine for a period of up to 2 hours due to the acidic environments.[12] These toxins act by inhibiting acetylcholinesterase and preventing acetylcholine from being hydrolyzed at the synapse, which allows acetylcholine to bind to membrane receptors. Subsequently animals undergo continuous muscle stimulation potentially leading to respiratory and brain hypoxia, in addition to convulsions and urinary incontinence.[11] Other SLUD like symptoms are common, and frequently seen clinical signs include muscle tremors, fasciculations, excessive salivation, and respiratory failure.[12,14] Since GNTs lack the ability to penetrate the blood–brain barrier, neurologic signs are limited to the periphery.[3] The LD_{50} in mice is 20 to 50 µg/kg via IP injection, with survival times of 10 to 30 minutes.[12,14]

β-methylaminoalanine

β-methylaminoalanine (BMAA) is an amino acid originally isolated from tropical cycad, and is produced by both diatoms/dinoflagellates and cyanobacteria found in fresh and salt water bodies.[3] BMAA is water soluble and can accumulate in seafood, as well as plants that were exposed to contaminated soil in experimental conditions. It acts as a glutamate agonist causing excitotoxicity in neurons. Additionally, it can cross the blood–brain barrier and causes depolarization of postsynaptic neurons leading to postsynaptic swelling and neuronal degeneration due to the influx of calcium.[3] Although controversial, it is also suspected of inciting protein misfolding and aggregation, neuroinflammation, and enzyme inhibition leading to neurodegenerative diseases such as amyotrophic lateral sclerosis (ALS), Alzheimer's, and Parkinson's disease in humans.[3] Specifically related to horses, it has been suggested as a possible cause of Equine Motor Neuron disease (EMN), though more research is needed to validate this claim.[15] The suspected pathophysiology is that overgrowth of naturally occurring cyanobacteria in the gut which produce BMAA occurs due to either a disease state or malnutrition, eventually affecting the brain.[15] In lab rodent studies, doses ranging from 500 mg/kg/day to 1000 mg/kg/day via IP injections showed degenerative changes of several cell populations in the cerebellar cortex. In macaques, oral doses from 100 mg/kg/day to 315 mg/kg/day showed neurologic impairment consistent with both upper and lower motor neurons, as well as the extrapyramidal system.[3]

CLINICAL SIGNS

Clinical signs vary, and their severity is directly related to the dose received. While there are very few case reports of blue green algae toxicosis in equines, **Table 1** provides an overview of the general clinical signs that are expected to occur with ingestion of a toxic dose.

DIAGNOSTICS

Necropsies of animals with suspected blue green algae toxicosis should be performed as soon as possible to avoid autolysis from interfering with test results.[17] If the necropsy cannot be performed in a timely fashion, the body should be stored under refrigerated conditions, and should not be frozen as this too will interfere with microscopic evaluation of tissues. Once samples have been obtained, they can be stored up to a month at $-20°C$, or for 3 months at $-80°C$.[17] Samples obtained from the live animal of a suspected blue green algae toxicosis should include stomach contents, serum, and urine. At least 100 g of gastric lavage material should be obtained prior to any adsorbants such as activated charcoal, and at least 20 mL of urine should be obtained.[17,18] Five mL of serum at a minimum should also be collected in a red top tube. Samples collected from dead animals should include a complete set of fresh and formalinized fixed tissue, including GI contents and urine (see Lynne Cassone's article, "Diagnostic Pathology of Equine Toxicoses," in this issue).[17,18] The tissues should be fixed in 10% neutral buffered formalin at approximately 10 times the volume of the tissue, though if excess volume is a shipping concern less formalin can be used once samples have fixed for at least 24 hours.[17] It should be noted that tissue testing is minimally offered, and potentially cost-prohibitive in many cases.

Water samples can also be used to confirm the presence of cyanotoxin-producing blue green algae. An example of a water sample submitted to a diagnostic laboratory can be seen in **Fig. 3**. Ideally, 1 L of water should be obtained and placed into a brown glass container, although plastic bottles wrapped in aluminum foil with secured fasteners are also acceptable.[17] A second 500 mL sample should also be obtained and diluted with 10% neutral buffered formalin. The second sample should consist of 500 mL of sampled water and 500 mL of formalin for a total of 1 L in similar packaging.[17] Gloves should be used when collecting a sample to avoid any possible skin irritation, and visible mats or scum should be included in water samples if applicable.

TREATMENT

Treatment overall is largely symptomatic as there is no antidote for blue green algae toxicosis.[19] Animals should be removed from the suspected source as soon as possible and given fresh water, and it should be noted that once clinical signs are observed GI decontamination is less likely to be therapeutic as enough toxin has already been absorbed to cause the clinical syndrome.[3,20] Ultimately, owners should be prepared that most animals affected have a poor prognosis. **Table 2** provides an overview of treatment based on the cyanotoxin the animal has been exposed to.

CONTROL

Preventative control is the best method to ensure the health of any animals against blue green algae toxicosis. As such, surface water should be monitored, especially in the later summer months where water temperatures can exceed 70°F and there

Table 1
Cyanotoxin overview

Cyanotoxin	Toxin Classification	Clinical Symptom	Acute LD$_{50}$ Dose (µG/KG; IP Injection in Mice)	Method of Action
Microcystin	Hepatotoxin	Intrahepatic shock, intrahepatic hemorrhage, severe hypoglycemia, elevated liver enzymes, elevated bilirubin, elevated bile acids, elevated blood urea nitrogen (BUN), elevated creatinine, pale mucous membranes, tachycardia, tachypnea, anorexia, abdominal pain, diarrhea, coma, possible hepatogenous photosensitivity	25–1000	Selective uptake by the liver via bile acid transporters; lesser uptake by the kidneys and central nervous system; inhibition of serine/threonine protein phosphatase 2 A
Nodularin	Hepatotoxin	Intrahepatic shock, intrahepatic hemorrhage, severe hypoglycemia, elevated liver enzymes, elevated bilirubin, elevated bile acids, elevated BUN, elevated creatinine, pale mucous membranes, tachycardia, tachypnea, anorexia, abdominal pain, diarrhea, coma	30–50	Selective uptake by the liver via bile acid transporters; lesser uptake by the kidneys and central nervous system; inhibition of serine/threonine protein phosphatase 2 A
Cylindrospermopsin	Hepatotoxin primarily; lesser renal toxin	Lethargy, anorexia, loss of body weight; marked delay in gastric emptying; Swollen/fatty liver, distended gall bladder, intestinal serosal hemorrhage, mottled/pale liver; pale, swollen kidney	200–2100	Inhibition of protein synthesis

(continued on next page)

Table 1
(continued)

Cyanotoxin	Toxin Classification	Clinical Symptom	Acute LD$_{50}$ Dose (µG/KG; IP Injection in Mice)	Method of Action
Anatoxin-a	Neurotoxin	Convulsion, muscle twitching, paralysis, respiratory failure, visual disturbances	250	Postsynaptic, depolarizing neuromuscular blockers
Saxitoxin	Neurotoxin	Vomiting, diarrhea, excessive sweating, salivation, headache	10–30	Sodium channel blocker
Guanitoxin	Neurotoxin	Convulsions, urinary distress, salivation, lacrimation, defecation	40	Acetylcholinesterase inhibitor
β-methylaminoalanine	Neurotoxin	Myoclonus, convulsions, uncontrolled urination/defecation[16] UMN and LMN signs	Unknown; presumptive 3 mg/g[16]	Glutamate receptor agonist; depolarization of postsynaptic neurons

Adapted from Beasley VR, Carmichael WW, Haschek WM, Colegrove KM, Solter PF. Phycotoxins. In: Elsevier EBooks;; 2023:305-391, Table 5.2; and Bláha L, Babica P, Maršálek B. Toxins produced in cyanobacterial water blooms - toxicity and risks. Interdisciplinary Toxicology. 2009;2(2), Table 2.

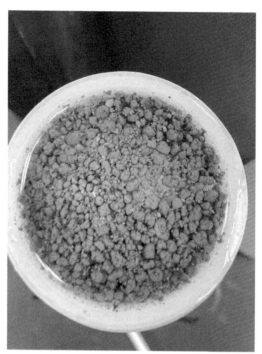

Fig. 3. An unusual gross appearance of microcystin submitted as a diagnostic case, note the globular appearance, these blooms can be very buoyant. (*Image courtesy*: Scott Fritz.)

is less rainfall.[20] Animals should be prevented from accessing water that has visible algal blooms, and fertilizer run-off should be prevented due to the increased risks of eutrophication.[19,20] Similarly, fertilizer should not be applied next to ponds or other bodies of water that animals may use as a drinking source.[19] Automatic watering systems that promote water movement should be used, as moving water helps prevent bloom formation.[20] Additionally, any supplements containing blue green algae as an ingredient should be screened for potential cyanotoxin contamination, or not be supplied to animals at all.

CASE STUDY SUMMARY

The following outline is a case summary reported by Mittelman and colleagues (2016) in which an 8-year-old Holsteiner gelding ultimately died from suspected microcystin toxicosis from a contaminated feed supplement.

- An 8-year-old Holsteiner gelding was given a powdered blue-green algae cyanobacteria supplement for purported hoof health.
- The patient became obtunded but otherwise was neurologically normal. He had icteric oral mucous membranes, as well as biochemical abnormalities that consisted of increased triglycerides, total protein, lactate, and serum sorbitol dehydrogenase (SDH). Aspartate aminotransferase (AST), ammonia, gamma-glutamyl transferase (GGT), bile acids, total bilirubin, indirect bilirubin, and direct bilirubin were also increased. These findings were suggestive of hepatic disease and hepatic encephalopathy.

Table 2
Treatment overview

Cyanotoxin	Treatment
Cylindrospermopsins	Supportive therapy; IV fluids to correct electrolyte imbalances, acidosis, and hypovolemic shock[3]
Microcystin/Nodularins	Rapidly bathe any cyanobacterial mats off the hair coat to prevent ingestion through grooming; administer oral or intragastric cholestyramine to reduce absorption from the digestive tract, though if this is unavailable activated charcoal should be used. Both initial doses can be given with sorbitol cathartic to accelerate gut motility, toxin binding, and evacuation; IV fluids to correct electrolyte imbalances; Plasma and/or blood transfusion to replace clotting proteins and blood loss, respectively; rifampin and cyclosporin-A are sometimes recommended in order to counteract liver uptake and inflammation; silybin has been recommended to help promote increased liver function; horses showing signs of secondary photosensitization should be kept indoors[3]
Anatoxin-a	Usually lethal and most animals die before supportive treatment can be initiated[3]; Diazepam given IV every 30 min to control seizures: Adults at 20–50 mg, foals at 0.05–0.4 mg/kg[20]
Guanitoxin	Some animal can die minutes after ingestion; further ingestion should be prevented and detoxification of the GI tract via activated charcoal should be performed; administration of antimuscarinic agents such as atropine, or agents that do not cross the blood–brain barrier such as glycopyrrolate can be used[3]
Saxitoxin	No known treatment
β-methylaminoalanine	No known treatment

- The feed supplement was determined to be positive for microcystin, and the horse was euthanized due to suspected microcystin toxicosis.
- AUS showed a gas extended stomach with a small liver.
- Two core liver biopsies revealed "periportal to midzonal hepatocellular necrosis characterized by cytoplasmic hypereosiniphilia and shrinkage with pyknosis and karyorrhexis."[21] The bile ducts were noted to be normal.
- Necropsy revealed a small liver with a flaccid, "dish rag" appearance. It was friable with orange-tan to green-brown parenchyma.
- Histopathology showed "severe periportal to massive necrosis with sinusoidal dilation and hemorrhage and relative sparing of centrilobular zones"[21]
  - Secondary changes included "early portal-portal bridging fibrosis, mild bile duct hyperplasia with canalicular cholestasis, and mild inflammation including lymphocytic periportal to midzonal infiltrates with scattered pigment-laden macrophages"[21]
  - Additional findings included "Alzheimer type II cells consistent with hepatic encephalopathy were present in the medulla, cerebellum, mesencephalon, diencephalon, and cerebral cortex",[21] and "mild eosinophilic colitis"[21] was also present.
- Algal testing via LC/MS revealed microcystin at 0.011 to 0.5 ppm in the supplement given to the gelding, as well as in 3 out of 5 remaining supplement containers.
  - Microcystin was not isolated in any of the tissue, blood, or GI contents tested.

CLINICS CARE POINTS

- Toxic dose data have not been developed for horses
- Cyanotoxins primarily affect the liver and nervous system of exposed animals
- Preventing exposure to contaminated water is imperative
- Diagnosis is primarily made utilizing clinical history, exposure to suspect water, histopathology, and detection of algae and/or toxins in water or gastric content
- There is no antidote for cyanotoxin exposure
- Cyanotoxins have zoonotic potential and care should be taken when working with suspect water sources

DISCLOSURE

The authors have no disclosures to make.

REFERENCES

1. Smith VH. Eutrophication. Elsevier EBooks.; 2009. p. 61–73. https://doi.org/10.1016/b978-012370626-3.00234-9.
2. Sha J, Xiong H, Liu C, et al. Harmful algal blooms and their eco-environmental indication. Chemosphere 2021;274:129912.
3. Beasley VR, Carmichael WW, Haschek WM, et al. Phycotoxins. London, UK: Elsevier EBooks.; 2023. p. 305–91.
4. Wolfe EM. Harmful algal bloom resources for livestock veterinarians. J Am Vet Med Assoc 2021;259(2):151–61.
5. Moreira C, Azevedo J, Antunes A, et al. Cylindrospermopsin: occurrence, methods of detection and toxicology. J Appl Microbiol 2012;114(3):605–20.
6. Yang Y, Yu G, Chen Y, et al. Four decades of progress in cylindrospermopsin research: The ins and outs of a potent cyanotoxin. J Hazard Mater 2021;406: 124653.
7. Roegner A, Brena BM, González-Sapienza G, et al. Microcystins in potable surface waters: toxic effects and removal strategies. J Appl Toxicol 2013;34(5): 441–57.
8. MacKeigan PW, Zastepa A, Taranu ZE, et al. Microcystin concentrations and congener composition in relation to environmental variables across 440 north-temperate and boreal lakes. Sci Total Environ 2023;884:163811.
9. Bouaïcha N, Miles CO, Beach DG, et al. Structural diversity, characterization and toxicology of microcystins. Toxins 2019;11(12):714.
10. Chen G, Wang L, Wang M, et al. Comprehensive insights into the occurrence and toxicological issues of nodularins. Mar Pollut Bull 2021;162:111884.
11. Christensen VG, Khan E. Freshwater neurotoxins and concerns for human, animal, and ecosystem health: A review of anatoxin-a and saxitoxin. Sci Total Environ 2020;736:139515.
12. Fernandes KA, Ferraz HG, Vereau F, et al. Availability of Guanitoxin in Water Samples Containing Sphaerospermopsis torques-reginae Cells Submitted to Dissolution Tests. Pharmaceuticals 2020;13(11):402.
13. Fiore MF, Lima SA, Carmichael WW, et al. Guanitoxin, re-naming a cyanobacterial organophosphate toxin. Harmful Algae 2020;92:101737.

14. Mahmood NHN, Carmichael WW. The pharmacology of anatoxin-a(s), a neurotoxin produced by the freshwater cyanobacterium Anabaena flos-aquae NRC 525-17. Toxicon 1986;24(5):425–34.

15. Brenner SR. Blue-green algae or cyanobacteria in the intestinal micro-flora may produce neurotoxins such as Beta-N-Methylamino-l-Alanine (BMAA) which may be related to development of amyotrophic lateral sclerosis, Alzheimer's disease and Parkinson-Dementia-Complex in humans and Equine Motor Neuron Disease in Horses. Med Hypotheses 2013;80(1):103.

16. Al-Sammak MA, Rogers DG, Hoagland KD. Acute β-N-Methylamino-L-alanine Toxicity in a Mouse Model. J Toxicol 2015;2015:1–9.

17. Iowa State University Veterinary Diagnostic Lab. Collection of Samples from Cyanobacterial Intoxications in Pets and Livestock. vetmed.iastate.edu. Available at: https://vetmed.iastate.edu/sites/default/files/vdpam/CyHABssamplecollection.pdf. Accessed July 20, 2023.

18. Office of Environmental Health Hazard Assessment (OEHHA), California Department of Public Health (CDPH). Blue Green Algae: A Veterinarian Reference. mywaterquality.ca.gov. Accessed July 20, 2023. https://mywaterquality.ca.gov/habs/what/vet_habs_factsheet.pdf.

19. Wilson DA. Clinical veterinary advisor: the horse. St. Louis, MO: Saunders; 2012.

20. Hovda LR, Benson D, Poppenga RH. Blackwell's five-minute veterinary consult clinical companion: equine toxicology. Hoboken, NJ: John Wiley & Sons; 2021.

21. Mittelman NS, Engiles JB, Murphy L, et al. Presumptive iatrogenic Microcystin-Associated liver failure and encephalopathy in a Holsteiner gelding. J Vet Intern Med 2016;30(5):1747–51.

Snake Envenomation

Lyndi L. Gilliam, DVM, PhD

KEYWORDS

- Snake • Pit viper • Antivenom • Snakebite • Envenomation • Vaccine • Horse

KEY POINTS

- Snakebite envenomation can be life-threatening.
- Antivenom is the mainstay of treatment for snakebite.
- The rattlesnake vaccine will not eliminate the need for veterinary care of snakebite but may reduce severity or delay onset of clinical signs with some snakes.

INTRODUCTION

Snakebite envenomation (SBE) in horses can have devastating outcomes. Little peer-reviewed literature regarding SBE in North American horses exists and published mortality rates are highly variable.[1] The mortality rate in horses is substantially higher than that reported in humans[2] but similar to dogs.[1] Venomous snakes inhabit 46 of the 50 United States (**Table 1**).[3] Being familiar with the venomous snakes in your area and the mechanisms of action of their venom components will promote rapid recognition of clinical signs of SBE and more treatment success. Although equine SBE research remains sparse, treatment has progressed with increased availability of veterinary antivenoms (AVs) and advances in critical care.

NORTH AMERICAN VENOMOUS SNAKES

Snakes in the family Viperidae subfamily Crotalinae are responsible for approximately 98% of indigenous human snakebites reported to poison control centers.[4] These snakes, commonly called pit vipers due to heat-sensing pits between their eyes and nostrils that allow them to sense prey, include rattlesnakes, copperheads, and water moccasins (**Figs. 1–6**).[5] Pit vipers have elliptical-shaped pupils, retractable fangs, and a unique diamond-shaped head due to venom glands on the sides of their heads.[5] In humans, copperheads contribute to 45% to 50% of yearly envenomations, rattlesnakes 30% to 40%, and water moccasins 10% to 15%.[4,6] Mortality is higher in humans, dogs, and cats bitten with rattlesnakes versus copperheads or water moccasins.[4] Because owners rarely witness their horse being bitten, mortality rate

College of Veterinary Medicine, Oklahoma State University, 2065 West Farm Road, Stillwater, OK 74078, USA
E-mail address: l.gilliam@okstate.edu

Vet Clin Equine 40 (2024) 133–150
https://doi.org/10.1016/j.cveq.2023.08.003
0749-0739/24/© 2023 Elsevier Inc. All rights reserved.

Table 1
North American pit vipers and their general geographic distribution

Common Name	Scientific Name	Distribution
Eastern Diamondback rattlesnake	Crotalus adamanteus	North Carolina, South Carolina, Georgia, Alabama, Mississippi, Louisiana, Florida
Western Diamondback rattlesnake	Crotalus atrox	California, Nevada, Arizona, New Mexico, Texas, Oklahoma, Arkansas
Mojave Desert Sidewinder	Crotalus cerastes	California, Nevada, Arizona, Utah
Midget Faded rattlesnake	Crotalus concolor	Wyoming, Utah, Colorado
Timber rattlesnake	Crotalus horridus	Texas, Oklahoma, Arkansas, Missouri, Tennessee, Kentucky, North Carolina, South Carolina, Georgia, Alabama, Mississippi, Louisiana, Florida, Pennsylvania, New Jersey, Maryland, Delaware, New York, New England, Virginia, West Virginia, Illinois, Indiana, Ohio, Minnesota, Wisconsin, Iowa, Nebraska
Rock rattlesnake	Crotalus lepidus	Arizona, New Mexico, Texas
Speckled rattlesnake	Crotalus mitchelli	California, Nevada, Arizona
Black-tailed rattlesnake	Crotalus molossus	Arizona, New Mexico, Texas
Twin-spotted rattlesnake	Crotalus pricei	Arizona
Mojave rattlesnake	Crotalus scutulatus	Nevada, SW Texas, South California, Tuscon to Phoenix Arizona, New Mexico
Red Diamond rattlesnake	Crotalus ruber	Washington, Oregon, Idaho
Tiger rattlesnake	Crotalus tigris	Arizona
Western rattlesnake	Crotalus viridis	Oregon, Idaho, Arizona, New Mexico, Texas, Montana, South Dakota, North Dakota, Nebraska, Iowa, Utah, Colorado, Kansas, Oklahoma
Prairie rattlesnake	Crotalus viridis viridis	Oregon, Idaho, Arizona, New Mexico, Texas, Montana, South Dakota, North Dakota, Nebraska, Iowa, Utah, Colorado, Kansas, Oklahoma, Wyoming, Alberta Canada
Grand Canyon rattlesnake	Crotalus viridis abyssus	Arizona

Southern Pacific rattlesnake	*Crotalus viridis helleri*	California
Great Basin rattlesnake	*Crotalus viridis lutosus*	Oregon, Idaho, California, Nevada, Arizona, Utah
Northern Pacific rattlesnake	*Crotalus viridis oreganus*	Washington, Oregon, Idaho, California, Nevada
Ridge-nosed rattlesnake	*Crotalus willardi*	Arizona
Massasauga rattlesnake	*Sistrurus catenatus*	Arizona, New Mexico, Texas, Michigan, Wisconsin, Minnesota, Nebraska, Iowa, Colorado, Kansas, Oklahoma, Arkansas, Missouri, Illinois, Indiana, Ohio, New York, Pennsylvania
Pigmy rattlesnake	*Sistrurus miliarius*	Texas, Oklahoma, Arkansas, Missouri, Tennessee, Florida, North Carolina, South Carolina, Georgia, Alabama, Mississippi, Louisiana
Southern Copperhead	*Agkistrodon contortrix*	Kansas, Oklahoma, Arkansas, Missouri, Tennessee, Kentucky, Illinois, Indiana, Ohio, North Carolina, South Carolina, Georgia, Alabama, Mississippi, Louisiana, Pennsylvania, New Jersey, Maryland, Delaware, Virginia, West Virginia, New York, New England
Eastern/Western Cottonmouth	*Agkistrodon piscivorus*	Texas, Oklahoma, Arkansas, Missouri, Tennessee, Kentucky, Illinois, North Carolina, South Carolina, Georgia, Alabama, Mississippi, Louisiana, Virginia, Iowa, Nebraska, Kansas

Data from Singletary EM, Rochman AS, Bodmer JC, Hostege CP. Envenomations. The Medical Clinics of North America 2005;89:1205 and Russell, FE. Snake Venom Poisoning in the United States. Ann. Rev. Med. 1980;31:250-251.

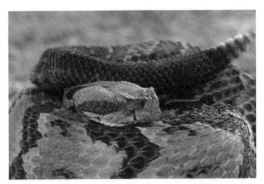

Fig. 1. *Crotalus horridus*—Timber rattlesnake—note thick, solid dark tail characteristic of timber rattlesnake. (*Photo courtesy* of John N. Gilliam, DVM, MS, DACVIM, DABVP. *From:* Gilliam LL, Brunker J. North American Snake Envenomation in the Dog and Cat. *Vet Clin North Am Small Anim Pract.* 2011;41(6):1239-1259. doi:10.1016/j.cvsm.2011.08.008, with permission.)

differences among pit viper SBE in horses is unknown. Rattlesnake bites are the most common SBE reported in the equine literature.

Pit vipers have a refined venom apparatus and can control how much venom they inject. Clinical signs of SBE are widely variable as they correlate with anatomic location of bite, status of the bite victim, and venom dose delivered. "Dry" or defensive bites, where little to no venom was injected, may cause minimal to no swelling compared with offensive or agonal bites which often involve delivery of large doses of venom resulting in severe tissue damage and systemic illness.[5] Pit viper venoms are similar but not identical and clinical signs may vary depending on the individual snake involved.

CLINICAL SIGNS OF ENVENOMATION

Snake venom is a complex mixture of enzymatic and nonenzymatic proteins that is intended to immobilize or kill prey and aid in digestion of prey swallowed whole.

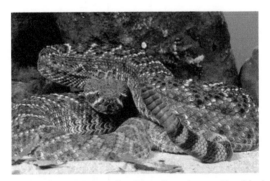

Fig. 2. *Crotalus atrox*—Western Diamondback rattlesnake—notice black and white bands on the tail, sometimes referred to as the coontail rattlesnake. (*Photo courtesy* of Dr. Charlotte L. Ownby. *From:* Gilliam LL, Brunker J. North American Snake Envenomation in the Dog and Cat. Vet Clin North Am Small Anim Pract. 2011;41(6):1239-1259. doi:10.1016/j.cvsm.2011.08.008, with permission.)

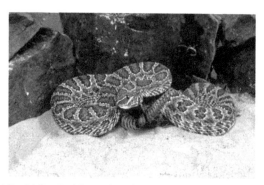

Fig. 3. *Crotalus viridis viridis*—Prairie rattlesnake. (Photo courtesy of Dr. Charlotte L. Ownby. *From*: Gilliam LL, Brunker J. North American Snake Envenomation in the Dog and Cat. *Vet Clin North Am Small Anim Pract*. 2011;41(6):1239-1259. doi:10.1016/j.cvsm.2011.08.008, with permission.)

Each clinical sign of SBE results from actions of one or a combination of several venom components. The severity of clinical signs depends not only on venom dose and type but also on patient-specific factors (age, size/weight, health status at time of bite, location of bite, and post-bite excitement/exercise).[5]

Visible snake fang puncture wounds are helpful in diagnosing SBE; however, absence of these wounds does not rule it out. If puncture wounds are located but clinical signs are minimal 1-hour post-bite, it is unlikely significant envenomation occurred (Mojave [MR] rattlesnake may be an exception).[7,8] Puncture wounds may be oozing due to coagulopathy making them easier to identify (**Fig. 7**), but in cases of "dry bite" or minimal envenomation, punctures may be difficult to find. In cases of severe SBE, marked swelling and tissue necrosis may obscure puncture wounds, especially if there is a delay to presentation post-bite.

Swelling secondary to SBE is painful and horses may resent having the area touched. Coagulopathy can result in frank hemorrhage and/or, in light-skinned horses, subcutaneous bruising at the bite site. Initially, swelling is edematous and inflamed and, with time, necrosis often occurs. Tissue damage is multifactorial with direct toxic

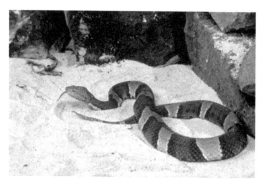

Fig. 4. Agkistrodon contortrix laticinctus—broad banded copperhead. (*Photo courtesy* of Charlotte Ownby. *From*: Gilliam LL, Brunker J. North American Snake Envenomation in the Dog and Cat. *Vet Clin North Am Small Anim Pract*. 2011;41(6):1239-1259. doi:10.1016/j.cvsm.2011.08.008, with permission.)

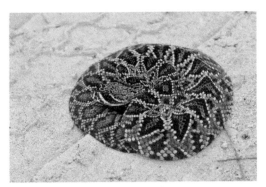

Fig. 5. *Crotalus adamanteus*—Eastern diamondback rattlesnake. (*Photo courtesy* of Dane Conley.)

effects of venom and indirect damage from profound swelling and the inflammatory response. Muzzle bites are most common, and as horses are obligate nasal breathers, profound swelling in response to SBE can result in respiratory distress and asphyxia (**Fig. 8**).

Tissue damage and necrosis is more severe with most rattlesnakes compared with copperhead or water moccasin bites.[9] Venom metalloproteinases (VMPs), hyaluronidase, serine proteinases, and phospholipases (VPLAs) are responsible for pain, tissue swelling, damage, and necrosis.[2,10] VMPs damage microvasculature leading to hemorrhage and cleave pro-tumor necrosis factor alpha (TNFα) releasing activated TNFα. Activated TNFα causes release of endogenous metalloproteinases resulting in a cyclical and uncontrolled inflammatory process.[10] VPLAs and VMPs were implicated as a cause of laminitis in horses bitten by a pit viper (*Bothrops sp*).[11] Laminitis has been reported in SBE horses in Colorado,[12] Texas, and Oklahoma (Scott Martin, DVM, Spearman, TX, personal communication, July 2023, Melanie Denton, DVM, Hollis, OK, Personal communication, July 2023). Although uncommon, laminitis is a risk in SBE horses as North American snake venoms do contain VMPs and VPLAs.

Coagulopathy is widely reported in humans and small animals secondary to SBE but is less well-defined in horses. Thrombocytopenia, prolonged prothrombin time (PT), and partial thromboplastin time (PTT) as well as spontaneous bleeding from the eyes, ears, nose, injection sites, or tracheotomy site have been reported in SBE

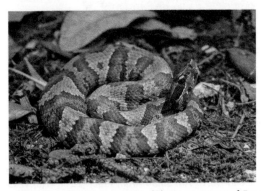

Fig. 6. *Agkistrodon piscivorus*—Water moccasin. (*Photo courtesy* of Dane Conley.)

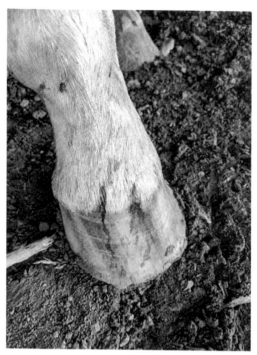

Fig. 7. Bite site with persistent hemorrhage on a distal limb. (*Photo courtesy* of Dr. Melanie Denton.)

horses.[12,13] Snake venom-induced coagulopathy is multifactorial. VMPs and other procoagulant factors consume coagulation factors and cause a venom-induced consumptive coagulopathy (VICC).[2] Venom fibrinolysins and thrombin-like enzymes destroy fibrin and fibrinogen resulting in defibrination and production of weak dysfunctional clots.[10] Disseminated intravascular coagulation (DIC) is rare following SBE but venom-induced defibrination may appear clinically similar to DIC.[10] Unlike DIC, venom defibrination patients may have normal platelet counts and no clinical bleeding.[10] Venom phospholipase A2s (VPLA2s) bind to phospholipids preventing activation of Factor X resulting in a dysfunctional clotting cascade and prolonged PT/PTT.[14] Venom can also cause thrombocytopenia or platelet dysfunction.[9] The exact mechanism of venom-induced thrombocytopenia is not known. At least two toxins (catrocollastatin—Western Diamondback [WD] rattlesnake, Crovidisin—prairie rattlesnake) have been identified that directly cause platelet dysfunction.[15,16] SBE horses can have a normal platelet number but abnormal platelet function.

Traditional coagulation assays (PT, PTT, D-dimer) are useful, but viscoelastic testing (thromboelastography [TEG], rotational thromboelastometry) gives a complete assessment of the entire coagulation process. In SBE dogs, TEG has been useful in directing AV treatment, and a hypocoagulable TEG tracing was associated with increased mortality.[17,18] In SBE horses TEG is useful in determining coagulation status and guiding AV dosing (Todd C. Holbrook, DVM, DACVIM, DACVSMR, Gainesville, FL, personal communication, July 2023) and is now available as a stall-side test.[a]

---

[a] VCM Vet™, Entegrion, Durham, NC.

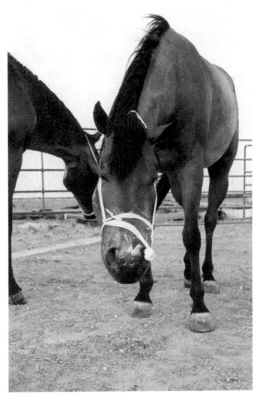

Fig. 8. Marked muzzle/head swelling post-rattlesnake bite, syringe casing placed to attempt to maintain airway.

Severe neurotoxicity is not widely reported in SBE horses in North America, but there are endemic snakes (Timber [TR], MR, Canebrake) with neurotoxic venom. MR envenomation can result in weakness, ataxia, flaccid paralysis, and respiratory failure due to an inhibition of calcium channels in the presynaptic motor neuron at the neuromuscular junction preventing acetylcholine release and thus muscular contraction.[10] These neurologic signs will not respond to calcium treatment,[10] and AV may be relatively ineffective at reversing them. Administering AV before neurologic signs appear is crucial. Neurotoxicity of MR venom is variable depending on location with those located near southwestern Arizona and southeastern California being more neurotoxic than those near Phoenix.[5]

Neurotoxicity caused by TR venom presents as fine, wave-like movements below the skin (myokymia). Venom toxins such as myotoxin a act on ion channels in muscle fibers causing skeletal muscle contracture. Calcium seems to be helpful in these cases.[10]

Pit viper venom-induced hypotension is likely multifactorial. WD rattlesnake venom contains a myocardial depressor protein that could result in hypotension.[19] Profound vasodilation leading to hypotension may occur in response to bradykinin (released by venom kininogenases) and prostaglandins (synthesized after phospholipid degradation by phospholipases A2 [PLA2s]).[20] Hypotension due to systemic hemorrhage and blood loss is rare in horses but could occur. Systemic increases in vascular permeability can contribute to fluid losses, hypovolemia, and hypotension. Hypotension can be more difficult to recognize in horses so measuring noninvasive blood pressure in envenomed horses may prove beneficial. Other measures of perfusion such as lactate may be beneficial if blood pressure monitoring is not available. If blood pressure does not improve with AV therapy and fluid resuscitation, pressors should be considered.[21]

Myocardial damage has been documented in some SBE horses, but there seem to be regional differences in the cardiotoxicity of rattlesnake venoms.[12,13,22] Persistent tachycardia and cardiac arrhythmias may be signs of myocardial damage.[12,13,22] The mechanism of myocardial damage is not well understood.

Acute kidney injury secondary to envenomation can occur and may be multifactorial. Hypotension or thrombotic microangiopathy may lead to renal hypoperfusion or ischemia. Myoglobin and hemoglobin released due to venom effects on muscle and red blood cells (RBCs) can result in a pigment nephropathy. There may also be direct cytotoxic damage to kidney tubular cells.

Regional lymphadenopathy may be noted near the bite site on careful physical examination. This should not be confused with infection as venom travels via lymphatics and may result in lymph node enlargement.[23] Lymphatic damage may also occur resulting in decreased lymphatic function and residual swelling, particularly in distal limb bites.[10]

EMERGENCY FIELD TREATMENT

Establishing an airway is a critical first step in SBE treatment of horses with bites to the head because of asphyxiation risk in these obligate nasal breathers. Owners can be instructed how to maintain a patent airway until veterinary care can be delivered by inserting a tube into the nare. A pliable tube (5/8–3/4 in diameter) with softened edges measuring the distance from the medial canthus of the eye to the nare (**Fig. 9**) can be placed up the ventral meatus and secured in place with tape. Owners should use caution as horses may be refractory to tube placement due to excruciating pain and if placed dorsally the tube could hit the ethmoid turbinates resulting in epistaxis.

If a horse is bitten in a remote location, driving a trailer to the horse would be beneficial. Increasing the horse's heart rate by walking may increase venom circulation. The horse should be kept as quiet as possible.

Field treatments proven ineffective and/or harmful that should not be used include cryotherapy, bite site incision and suction, hot packs, electrical shock therapy, and tourniquets.[5] Tourniquets are controversial. It is widely agreed on that arterial tourniquets should not be used with pit viper envenomation due to the venom and inflammatory mediator bolus that can occur when they are removed.[5,6,10] Although some compression wraps have shown benefit with coral snake envenomation,[24] evidence is lacking of their benefit in pit viper envenomation. If a horse presents with a tourniquet in place, a slow release of pressure should be performed. A looser tourniquet is placed above the initial tourniquet before it is released and this process of gradually decreasing the pressure is continued over 15 to 20 minutes, ideally while administering AV.[25]

Time to treatment is an important prognostic indicator in SBE patients.[6,26] The most important goal should be getting the horse to veterinary treatment as soon as possible. Owners should not delay or risk getting bitten to identify the snake but could move out of striking distance and take a quick picture when feasible.[27] Agonal bites result in release of significant amounts of venom so attempting to kill the snake and increasing the risk of being bitten is ill-advised.[5]

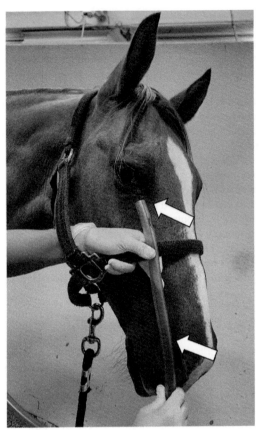

Fig. 9. Ideal length of tube passed up the ventral meatus to maintain airway patency, measuring from medial canthus of eye to nare (*white arrows*). (*Photo courtesy* of Dr. Brittnee Sayler.)

DIAGNOSTIC TESTING

Routine hematology, blood chemistry, and coagulation testing are helpful in SBE cases. Nonspecific hemogram changes may include hemoconcentration or anemia, leukocytosis more commonly than leukopenia, and thrombocytopenia.[12,13] Manual review of a blood smear allows for a manual platelet count because machine counts are often affected by platelet clumping in horses and RBC morphology assessment. The exposure of equine RBCs to WD rattlesnake venom resulted in dose-dependent changes in RBC morphology (low venom concentration = Type I and II echinocytes, increasing venom concentrations = Type III echinocytes, spheroechinocytes, spherocytes)[28] suggesting this could be an indicator of venom dose but in vivo documentation is lacking. The absence of echinocytes does not rule out envenomation.[28] TEG gives a more complete picture of coagulation but, if unavailable, activated clotting time, PT, PTT, D-dimer, and fibrinogen are helpful. In humans, a 20-minute whole blood clotting test has been useful.[29] In horses, a clot should form in a glass red top tube within 30 minutes. Performing a normal control with the snakebite patient could give a crude idea of the presence of coagulopathy. Hypocoagulability is the most common finding with SBE, and fibrinogen is more commonly normal or low.[9]

Both myotoxin a and VPLA2s in pit viper venoms disrupt calcium regulation within skeletal muscle cells resulting in increased intracellular calcium and subsequent muscle damage with resultant increases in creatine phosphokinase and aspartate aminotransferase.[20,30] Skeletal muscle may also be damaged by reduced perfusion in the bite area,[31] or if direct intramuscular injection occurs, venom proteolytic enzymes will damage muscle fibers.[6]

Hypokalemia is the primary electrolyte abnormality observed with pit viper envenomation.[5] Potassium supplementation may be needed as its depletion can lead to myocardial dysfunction.

Azotemia may be noted in SBE horses. Performing a urinalysis is useful to look for pigmenturia and help determine if azotemia is prerenal or renal. Renal damage is more often secondary to poor perfusion or pigmenturia than primary venom damage.[31]

Careful cardiac auscultation following SBE is crucial. Horses should be auscultated for a full minute several times a day to attempt to detect any abnormal rhythms. In horses with persistent tachycardia or suspected abnormal rhythm, electrocardiogram (ECG) should be performed. Cardiac troponin I (cTnI) should be considered in rattlesnake bitten horses, especially if any abnormalities are auscultated. A onetime measurement may not be adequate to detect myocardial damage as peak increase may not be seen for several days post-bite.[22] One sample should be taken within the first 24 hours and if abnormal it should be rechecked every 24 hours until it is no longer increasing. If the first sample is normal, it should be checked again at 48 hours and 1 week to be certain an increase is not observed. Signs of cardiac disease may not occur for several months after SBE resulting in the risk of horses being back in work without knowing they have abnormal myocardial function. Measuring cTnI can detect myocardial inflammation and prompt a thorough cardiac evaluation before a horse is put back in work. Full echocardiogram should be performed in horses with moderate to marked increases in cTnI, persistent tachycardia, or any other signs of cardiac dysfunction before returning to work. cTnI is relatively stable and samples can be shipped refrigerated for analysis.

Determining the progression of envenomation can be helpful in patient assessment as well as monitoring treatment efficacy. For head bites, it can be difficult to assess bite progression but the extent of the swelling can be marked and monitored every 30 minutes to determine if it is progressing caudally up the face. Circumferential measurements of the bite area can also be made, if the horse will allow, detecting progression. Ideally, the circumference of the bite area should be taken every 30 to 60 minutes until the measurement is static for four measurements and then two to three times daily for 48 hours to help assess progression of the bite.[5]

A rattlesnake bite severity scoring system (RBSS) has been developed for horses (**Table 2**).[13] This scoring system can be used as an objective determinant of bite severity, to aid in the decision to administer AV and to track progression of the bite.

IN-HOSPITAL TREATMENT

If a horse arrives in respiratory distress and a nasal tube cannot be placed, a tracheostomy will be needed. If signs of coagulopathy are present, administering AV before, or simultaneously with, tracheostomy may avoid excessive hemorrhage.

Once an airway is established, treatment involves supportive care and medications to decrease venom effects. Horses with head bites often cannot eat or drink for several days so hydration must be maintained with intravenous or rectal fluid administration. Serum triglycerides should be monitored in anorexic horses that are overweight, have a history of pars pituitary intermedia dysfunction or equine metabolic

Table 2
Rattlesnake-bite severity scoring system in horses

Variable	Score	Signs
Respiratory system	0	Unremarkable (8–20 breaths/minute)
	1	Mild signs of respiratory distress
	2	Tachypnea present and increased work of breathing
	3	Severe respiratory distress with or without cyanosis
Cardiovascular system	0	Unremarkable (32–50 beats/minute)
	1	Mild tachycardia (>50 but ≤60 beats/minute)
	2	Moderate tachycardia (>60 but ≤80 beats/minute) or blood lactate concentration ≥2.5 but ≤ 4.0 mmol/L
	3	Severe tachycardia (80 beats/minute) or blood lactate concentration >4 mmol/L
Wound appearance	0	No swelling
	1	Mild swelling involving only the nose or distal portion of the limb
	2	Moderate swelling involving entire head or distal portion of the limb
	3	Severe swelling spreading to the head or trunk
Hemostasis	0	No abnormalities
	1	PT and PTT higher than reference limit but <25% increase or <120,000 but ≥100,000 platelets/μL of blood
	2	PT and PTT >25% but ≤50% higher than reference limits or <100,000 but ≥50,000 platelets/μL of blood
	3	PT and PTT >50% higher than reference limits but ≤100% of the reference limits or <50,000 but ≥20,000 platelets/μL of blood
	4	PT and PTT >100% higher than reference limits or <20,000 platelets/μL of blood with signs of spontaneous bleeding

From Fielding CL, Pusterla N, Magdesian KG, Higgins JC, Meier CA. Rattlesnake envenomation in horses: 58 cases (1992–2009). *J Am Vet Med Assoc.* 2011;238(5):631-635. doi:10.2460/javma.238.5.631; with permission.

syndrome and donkeys, ponies or pony crosses. Feeding mashes can help horses eat, whereas their muzzle is painful and swollen.

SBE horses should be monitored for 8 hours minimum even if signs initially seem mild. The snakebite severity score (SBSS) should be calculated on presentation and again 6 hours post-presentation to ensure subtle progression is not occurring.[5]

AV is the mainstay of treatment for SBE. AVs can either be whole IgG or IgG that has had the Fc portion removed leaving either the intact F(ab')2 portion or single Fab portions making the product less likely to cause an adverse reaction. Having a larger molecular size, whole IgG AV products have lower volume of distribution, distribute slower into tissues, and are cleared slower from circulation.[32] Prolonged time in circulation may be beneficial in combatting venom components that remain in circulation longer or venom that is released into circulation once damaged, envenomed tissues are reperfused.[32] Compared with whole IgG products, F(ab)2' products are less likely to cause a reaction, have a larger volume of distribution, more rapidly distribute into tissues, and are more rapidly cleared from circulation.[32] Fab has the smallest molecular size, the largest volume of distribution, most rapid tissue distribution, and the most rapid clearance. Rapid clearance of F(ab)2' and Fab products can result in recurrence of envenomation signs and the need to repeat AV administration as often as every 6 hours.[32,33] Fortunately, great developments have made

AVs readily available for veterinary use. There is one whole IgG product[b] labeled for use in horses, cats, and dogs, and 1 F(ab)2'[c] product labeled for use in dogs. Both products are manufactured in horses so risk of adverse allergic reaction in horses is minimal. Research in horses receiving a whole IgG AV revealed zero adverse reactions, both short and long term.[34] Screening of equine donors for hepatitis viruses has minimized concerns of Theiler's disease when using equine origin products in horses. AV-containing antibodies to venom of the species of snake that caused the bite are ideal. The veterinary whole IgG[b] product is manufactured using North American pit viper venoms, but the F(ab)2'[c] product is not. Dosing AV is difficult because the dose needed depends on the unknown amount of venom delivered. An initial dose of AV (50 mL of equine labeled product[b]) can be given and then clinical signs monitored. If the horse is declining within 6 hours of AV administration or no improvement is seen in 24 hours, additional dosing should be considered. In other species, the RBSS is often used to determine the need for AV. Rattlesnake SBE does not always require AV in dogs,[35] and copperhead envenomation rarely requires AV for clinical sign resolution in people.[36] However, in rattlesnake SBE horses where cardiotoxicity, tissue necrosis and laminitis can be devastating, AV should be offered in any moderate to severe envenomation and any patient with increased cTnI. Early AV intervention results in improved outcomes.[27] AV will not eliminate all tissue damage but may reduce life-threatening systemic effects. Patients presenting greater than 24 hours post-bite with signs of envenomation may still have circulating venom and therefore benefit from AV treatment. For adverse AV reactions, the infusion should be stopped and then resumed at a slower rate once the horse stabilizes. To treat AV reactions in horses, steroids are most often given. Antihistamines can be used and rarely epinephrine is needed.

Snakebites are painful and analgesia in horses often centers on nonsteroidal antiinflammatory drugs. Although beneficial in blocking prostaglandins and providing analgesia, they may exert negative effects on platelets; however, in human copperhead SBE, detrimental coagulation effects were not seen with non-steroidal anti-inflammatory drug (NSAID) use.[37] Judicious use is recommended in coagulopathic horses, and alternate sources of analgesia should be considered such as opioids and/or lidocaine. Morphine-related histamine release, reported in other species, can mimic an AV reaction; therefore, fentanyl is preferred.[5]

Corticosteroids are controversial in snakebite therapy in humans and dogs but are widely used in treating horses. They are not recommended in human SBE treatment except in cases of adverse AV reactions.[38] Steroids have been shown to have some detrimental and some beneficial effects in envenomation models.[39] One retrospective study in horses concluded that short-term use of short-acting steroids may be beneficial but their prolonged use should be avoided.[12] Which corticosteroid and what dose is the most appropriate remain to be determined.[39]

Although venom has bacteriocidal activity, bacteria can be found in snake's mouths.[39] There are no prospective studies evaluating antimicrobial use in North American SBE horses. The inability to keep horse wounds free from contamination may warrant antibiotics in cases with tissue necrosis. Procaine penicillin has been associated with increased survival in SBE horses, and broad spectrum antimicrobials have been shown to be effective in treating dogs.[39,40] Clinician discretion should be used in determining which patients need antimicrobials.

---

[b] Rattler Antivenin™, Mg Biologics, Ames, IA.

[c] VenomVet™, MT Venom, LLC, Canoga Park, CA.

Dimethyl sulfoxide (DMSO) is widely used in equine medicine, and some practitioners report using it in SBE cases. The author does not recommend using topical DMSO in SBE cases due to the risk of increasing venom circulation. More evidence is needed to understand the role of systemic DMSO in SBE treatment.

PLA2s associated with envenomation cause coagulopathy, neurotoxicity, tissue damage, and pain. In an experimental coral snake SBE porcine model, 45 minutes post-venom administration AV was unable to reverse neurologic signs; however, neurotoxicity was completely reversed with administration of a PLA2 inhibitor, LY315920.[41] Phospholipase inhibitors are being investigated in human snakebite patients and are a promising future direction for equine snakebite.[42]

PROGNOSIS

Mortality following SBE in North America in horses ranges from 5% to 25%.[12,13,22] Snake type, venom dose, and post-bite care all affect prognosis. Cardiac damage, laminitis, or severe tissue necrosis involving distal limbs may result in a poor prognosis for return to athletic function. More data are needed on long-term prognosis of SBE horses.

PREVENTION

Vaccination for reduction of SBE-related morbidity is not a new concept. A *Bothrops asper* toxoid vaccine given to cattle prevented systemic signs and need for AV with low-dose venom and delayed onset of systemic signs with high dose venom but AV was still needed.[43] A rattlesnake toxoid vaccine[d] is available to reduce SBE morbidity. No in vivo efficacy studies have been performed in horses. Vaccine response is highly variable among horses, and vaccine titers are significantly lower than natural envenomation titers.[44] Inactivating venom results in a loss of epitopes responsible for the immunogenicity and may explain a weaker vaccine immune reponse.[44] Vaccine titers were not long-lasting in horses in one study[44] indicating the need for strategic vaccination with snakebite season. No adverse vaccine effects were noted in this study.[44] The vaccine is made using WD rattlesnake venom and relies on cross-reactivity for protection against other pit vipers. Some cross-reactivity may occur but will vary with species. In a mouse model, vaccinated mice had increased survival rates compared with non-vaccinated mice when challenged with WD rattlesnake venom, but there was a smaller difference in mice challenged with Northern Pacific rattlesnake venom and no difference in mice challenged with Southern Pacific rattlesnake venom.[45] The author's opinion is that in pit viper (particularly WD rattlesnake) endemic areas, the vaccine may offer benefit and should be considered. The vaccine will not likely eliminate the need for veterinary care of SBE but may lessen clinical signs or at least delay onset of clinical signs allowing more time to reach veterinary care. There have been anecdotal reports of anaphylaxis related to the rattlesnake vaccine in dogs.[46] The author is not aware of these reports in horses but it is worth consideration as SBE anaphylaxis occurs in humans.[47]

SUMMARY

SBE is an emergency and veterinary care should be sought quickly. AV is the mainstay of treatment and should be offered in any moderate to severe envenomation. The early

---

[d] Rattlesnake Vaccine (*Crotalus Atrox* Toxoid), Red Rock Biologics, Woodland, CA.

administration of AV improves prognosis. If signs of cardiac inflammation/damage are noted, thorough cardiac examination should be performed before returning the horse to work. Vaccination may be beneficial in some areas, but will not eliminate the need for veterinary care if a bite occurs. The risk of vaccine or venom anaphylaxis in vaccinated horses, although seemingly rare, should be discussed with the owner.

CLINICS CARE POINTS

- In coagulopathic snakebite envenomation (SBE) horses needing tracheotomy, administering antivenom before or during the tracheostomy may prevent excessive hemorrhage.
- Antivenom seems safe and effective in treating SBE in horses and should be considered a mainstay of treatment.
- Short duration, short-acting steroids may be beneficial but should not be used long term.
- The rattlesnake vaccine, if given, should be administered strategically with snakebite season.
- The rattlesnake vaccine will not offer protection for all pit viper bites and will not eliminate the need for veterinary care if a vaccinated horse is bitten, but may reduce or delay onset of clinical signs caused by some snakes.

ACKNOWLEDGMENTS

The author would like to acknowledge Jose M. Gutierrez for sharing his valuable expertise in reviewing this manuscript and Todd C. Holbrook and John N. Gilliam for their editorial assistance during manuscript preparation.

DISCLOSURE

The author has performed research without financial compensation for MgBiologics and Ophirex.

REFERENCES

1. Bolon I, Finat M, Herrera M, et al. Snakebite in domestic animals: First global scoping review. Prev Vet Med 2019;170:104729. https://doi.org/10.1016/j.prevetmed.2019.104729.
2. Seifert SA, Armitage JO, Sanchez EE. Snake Envenomation. In: Longo DL, editor. N Engl J Med 2022;386(1):68–78. https://doi.org/10.1056/NEJMra2105228.
3. Holder K. The 4 Main Types of Venomous Snakes in the United States. az animals. Available at: https://a-z-animals.com/blog/the-4-main-types-of-venomous-snakes-in-the-united-states/.
4. Greene SC, Folt J, Wyatt K, et al. Epidemiology of fatal snakebites in the United States 1989–2018. Am J Emerg Med 2021;45:309–16. https://doi.org/10.1016/j.ajem.2020.08.083.
5. Peterson ME. Snake Bite: Pit Vipers. Clin Tech Small Anim Pract 2006;21(4):174–82. https://doi.org/10.1053/j.ctsap.2006.10.008.
6. Gold B, Wingert W. Snake venom poisoning in the United States: a review of therapeutic practice. South Med J 1994;87:579–89.
7. Mansfield P. The management of snake venom poisoning in dogs. Compend Continuing Educ Pract Vet 1984;6:988–92.
8. Russell F. Snake venom poisoning in the United States. Annu Rev Med 1980;31:247–59.

9. Gilliam LL, Brunker J. North American Snake Envenomation in the Dog and Cat. Vet Clin North Am Small Anim Pract 2011;41(6):1239–59. https://doi.org/10.1016/j.cvsm.2011.08.008.

10. Holstege C, Miller M, Wermuth M, et al. Crotalid snake envenomation. Crit Care Clin 1997;13(4):889–921.

11. Acosta De Pérez O, Teibler P, Leiva L, et al. Equine laminitis: Bites by *Bothrops* spp cause hoof lamellar pathology in the contralateral as well as in the bitten limb. Toxicon 2006;48(3):307–12. https://doi.org/10.1016/j.toxicon.2006.06.010.

12. Dickinson CE, Traub-Dargatz JL, Dargatz DA, et al. Rattlesnake venom poisoning in horses: 32 cases (1973-1993). J Am Vet Med Assoc 1996;208(11):1866–71.

13. Fielding CL, Pusterla N, Magdesian KG, et al. Rattlesnake envenomation in horses: 58 cases (1992–2009). J Am Vet Med Assoc 2011;238(5):631–5. https://doi.org/10.2460/javma.238.5.631.

14. Ownby C, Bjarnason J, Tu A. Hemorrhagic toxins from rattlesnake (*Crotalus atrox*) venom. Pathogenesis of hemorrhage induced by three purified toxins. Am J Pathol 1978;93:201–18.

15. Zhou Q, Smith J, Grossman M. Molecular cloning and expression of catrocollastatin, a snake-venom protein from *Crotalus atrox* (wester diamondback rattlesnake) which inhibits platelet adhesion to collagen. Biochem J 1995;307(Pt 2):411–7.

16. Liu C, Huang T. Crovidisin, a colagen-binding protein isolated from snake venom of Crotalus viridis, prevents platelet-collagen interaction. Arch Biochem Biophys 1997;337:291–9.

17. Armentano RA, Bandt C, Schaer M, et al. Thromboelastographic evaluation of hemostatic function in dogs treated for crotalid snake envenomation: TEG in dogs treated for pit viper envenomation. J Vet Emerg Crit Care 2014;24(2):144–53. https://doi.org/10.1111/vec.12139.

18. Lieblick BA, Bergman PJ, Peterson NW. Thromboelastographic evaluation of dogs bitten by rattlesnakes native to southern California. Am J Vet Res 2018;79(5):532–7. https://doi.org/10.2460/ajvr.79.5.532.

19. Bonilla C, Rammel O. Comparative biochemistry and pharmacology of salivary gland secretions. III. Chromatographic isolation of a myocardial depressor protein (MDP) from the venom of *Crotalus atrox*. J Chromatogr 1976;124:304–14.

20. Hudelson S, Hudelson P. Pathophysiology of snake envenomation and evaluation of treatments: part 1. Compend Continuing Educ Pract Vet 1995;17:889–97.

21. WHO. Guidelines for the Management of snakebites. 2nd edition. New Delhi, India: World Health Organization; 2016.

22. Gilliam LL, Holbrook TC, Ownby CL, et al. Cardiotoxicity, Inflammation, and Immune Response after Rattlesnake Envenomation in the Horse. J Vet Intern Med 2012;26(6):1457–63. https://doi.org/10.1111/j.1939-1676.2012.01022.x.

23. Singletary E, Rochman A, Bodmer J, et al. Envenomations. Med Clin North Am 2005;89(6):1195–224.

24. Peterson ME. Snake Bite: Coral Snakes. Clin Tech Small Anim Pract 2006;21(4):183–6. https://doi.org/10.1053/j.ctsap.2006.10.005.

25. Bush SP, Kinlaw SB. Management of a Pediatric Snake Envenomation After Presentation With a Tight Tourniquet. Wilderness Environ Med 2015;26(3):355–8. https://doi.org/10.1016/j.wem.2015.01.005.

26. Hardy DS. Fatal rattlesnake envenomation in Arizona: 1969-1984. J Toxicol Clin Toxicol 1986;24.

27. Russell JJ, Schoenbrunner A, Janis JE. Snake Bite Management: A Scoping Review of the Literature. Plast Reconstr Surg - Glob Open. 2021;9(4):e3506. https://doi.org/10.1097/GOX.0000000000003506.

28. Walton R, Brown D, Hamar D, et al. Mechanisms of echinocytosis induced by *Crotalus atrox* venom. Vet Pathol 1997;34(5):442–9.

29. Lamb T, Abouyannis M, Oliveira SS de, et al. The 20-minute whole blood clotting test (20WBCT) for snakebite coagulopathy - A systematic review and meta-analysis of diagnostic test accuracy. PLoS Negl Trop Dis 2021; 15(8):1–20.

30. Tu A. Rattlesnake venoms: their actions and treatment. Marcel Dekker; 1982.

31. Hudelson S, Hudelson P. Pathophysiology of snake envenomation and evaluation of treatments: part II. Compend Continuing Educ Pract Vet 1995;17: 1035–40.

32. Carotenuto SE, Bergman PJ, Ray JR, et al. Retrospective comparison of three antivenoms for the treatment of dogs with crotalid envenomation. J Am Vet Med Assoc 2021;259(5):503–9. https://doi.org/10.2460/javma.259.5.503.

33. Boyer L, Seifert SA, Cain J. Recurrence phenomena after immunoglobulin therapy for snake envenomations: Part 2. Guidelines for clinical management with crotaline fab antivenom. Ann Emerg Med 2001;37(2):196–201.

34. Estrada R, Herrera M, Segura Á, et al. Intravenous administration of equine-derived whole IgG antivenom does not induce early adverse reactions in non-envenomed horses and cows. Biologicals 2010;38(6):664–9. https://doi.org/10.1016/j.biologicals.2010.08.002.

35. Hackett T, Wingfield W, Mazzaferro E, et al. Clinical findings associated with prairie rattlesnake bite in dogs: 100 cases (1989-1998). J Am Vet Med Assoc 2002; 220(11):1675–80.

36. Walker PJ, Morrison RL. Current Management of Copperhead Snakebite. J Am Coll Surg 2011;212(4):470–4. https://doi.org/10.1016/j.jamcollsurg.2010.12.049.

37. PHam HX, Mullins ME. Safety of nonsteroidal anti-inflammatory drugs in copperhead snakebite patients. Clin Toxicol 2018;56(11):1121–7.

38. Lavonas EJ, Ruha AM, Banner W, et al. Unified treatment algorithm for the management of crotaline snakebite in the United States: results of an evidence-informed consensus workshop. BMC Emerg Med 2011;11(1):2. https://doi.org/10.1186/1471-227X-11-2.

39. Armentano RA, Schaer M. Overview and controversies in the medical management of pit viper envenomation in the dog: Management of pit viper envenomation in the dog. J Vet Emerg Crit Care 2011;21(5):461–70. https://doi.org/10.1111/j.1476-4431.2011.00677.x.

40. Tirosh-Levy S, Solomovich-Manor R, Comte J, et al. *Daboia* (*Vipera*) palaestinae Envenomation in 123 Horses: Treatment and Efficacy of Antivenom Administration. Toxins 2019;11(3):168. https://doi.org/10.3390/toxins11030168.

41. Lewin M, Gilliam L, Gilliam J, et al. Delayed LY333013 (Oral) and LY315920 (Intravenous) Reverse Severe Neurotoxicity and Rescue Juvenile Pigs from Lethal Doses of *Micrurus fulvius* (Eastern Coral Snake) Venom. Toxins 2018;10(11): 479. https://doi.org/10.3390/toxins10110479.

42. Lewin MR, Carter RW, Matteo IA, et al. Varespladib in the Treatment of Snakebite Envenoming: Development History and Preclinical Evidence Supporting Advancement to Clinical Trials in Patients Bitten by Venomous Snakes. Toxins 2022;14(11):783. https://doi.org/10.3390/toxins14110783.

43. Herrera M, González K, Rodríguez C, et al. Active immunization of cattle with a bothropic toxoid does not abrogate envenomation by *Bothrops asper* venom,

but increases the likelihood of survival. Biologicals 2017;46:1–5. https://doi.org/10.1016/j.biologicals.2016.10.008.

44. Gilliam LL, Carmichael RC, Holbrook TC, et al. Antibody Responses to Natural Rattlesnake Envenomation and a Rattlesnake Toxoid Vaccine in Horses. Clin Vaccine Immunol 2013;20(5):732–7. https://doi.org/10.1128/CVI.00004-13.

45. Cates CC, Valore EV, Couto MA, et al. Comparison of the protective effect of a commercially available western diamondback rattlesnake toxoid vaccine for dogs against envenomation of mice with western diamondback rattlesnake (*Crotalus atrox*), northern Pacific rattlesnake (*Crotalus oreganus oreganus*), and southern Pacific rattlesnake (*Crotalus oreganus helleri*) venom. Am J Vet Res 2015;76(3):272–9. https://doi.org/10.2460/ajvr.76.3.272.

46. Gil BD. Activated immune mechanisms of the veterinary rattlesnake vaccine and its determination of adverse reactions in canine patients. The University of Arizona; 2022.

47. Ryan K, Caravati E. Life-threatening anaphylaxis following envenomation by two different species of Crotalidae. J Wilderness Med 1994;5(3):263–8.

Other toxicants

Therapeutic Medications and Illicit Medications and Supplements

Lynn Rolland Hovda, RPH, DVM, MS[a,b],*

KEYWORDS

- Stacking • Illicit medications • Illegally compounded medications
- Herbal supplements

KEY POINTS

- Combining multiple therapeutic medications especially if they are in the same class may cause a toxic reaction at lower doses.
- Illicit medications are often human products used off label or illegally compounded medications.
- Supplement labels should be read carefully, and any unknown substances investigated before use.

THERAPEUTIC MEDICATIONS
Introduction

The list of therapeutic medications associated with toxic reactions is lengthy and discussing each one in this article is not possible. The most common therapeutic medications with known toxic reactions are discussed, whereas rarely used drugs, for example, digoxin, atropine, and others, are not. The goal is to provide the best medical care while ensuring the safety and welfare of the horse. This makes understanding pharmacokinetics and the ultimate disposition of a medication a vital part of the treatment plan. The use of multiple medications makes this challenging. What might be an adverse reaction to a substance may become a toxicity when administered with other medications. Stacking, the coadministration of 2 or 3 medications in a similar class, can easily result in toxicity.

DISCUSSION
Antibiotics

Most presumed antibiotic-related toxicities are a dose-related continuation of an adverse effect and should be treated as such. The main exception is a drug in the

[a] Safetycall International and Pet Poison Helpline, 3600 American Boulevard West, Suite 725, Bloomington, MN 55431, USA; [b] Department of Veterinary and Biomedical Sciences, College of Veterinary Medicine, University of Minnesota, St. Paul, MN, USA
* Corresponding author. 3600 American Boulevard West, Suite 725, Minneapolis, MN 55431.
E-mail address: lhovda@safetycall.com

Vet Clin Equine 40 (2024) 151–160
https://doi.org/10.1016/j.cveq.2023.10.003
0749-0739/24/© 2023 Elsevier Inc. All rights reserved.

tetracycline group. Horses receiving intravenous (IV) oxytetracycline have collapsed from rapid administration, and the use in neonatal foals for flexural limb deformities has been associated with acute kidney injury.[1] Intravenous administration of doxycycline, regardless of the rate, is associated with cardiovascular (CV) abnormalities and death.[2] Changes in the gastrointestinal (GI) flora and the potential for enterocolitis have been associated with oxytetracycline but not oral doxycycline.

Antipsychotic Agents

Fluphenazine and reserpine are among the oldest antipsychotics used in horses. Injectable fluphenazine is available as human product; reserpine is compounded as injectable and oral. Fluphenazine crosses the blood–brain barrier (BBB) and antagonizes the dopamine D2 receptors; reserpine crosses the BBB and inhibits the uptake of dopamine, serotonin, and norepinephrine. The toxic dose is not well defined but toxicosis is associated with the use of 25 to 125 mg IV or IM fluphenazine[3–5] and 10 to 12.5 mg IM reserpine.[6,7] Clinical signs associated with fluphenazine toxicosis occur in 12 to 36 hours and in 5 to 6 hours with IM reserpine. Most striking are the neurologic signs including agitation, sweating, and abnormal behaviors such as striking, pawing, head tossing, and gait abnormalities. Other common signs include colic and profuse diarrhea, priapism, respiratory distress, and bradycardia. Typically, signs resolve in about 72 hours for fluphenazine and 48 hours for reserpine.

Other medications such as aripiprazole, fluoxetine, paroxetine, trazodone, and venlafaxine have been used to control behavior in horses. Of these, fluoxetine and trazodone, selective serotonin reuptake inhibitors, are used the most. No adverse or toxic reactions were noted in horses receiving fluoxetine at 0.25 mg/kg PO q 24 hours for 8 weeks.[8] It is difficult to state whether horses dosed higher than 0.25 to 0.5 mg/kg would develop serotonin syndrome because no toxicologic studies have been published.[8] Trazadone dosed orally at 4 mg/kg provided acceptable sedation in one study[9] while horses in a second study receiving 10 mg/kg developed oversedation, ataxia, arrhythmias, muscle fasciculations, and body temperature changes.[10,11]

Intravenous trazadone is contraindicated due to the rapid onset of aggression and excitability.[9,11]

Bronchodilators

The most common bronchodilators used in horses are clenbuterol, which is Food and Drug Administration (FDA) approved for oral use in horses, and albuterol, which is used off label. Both are beta-2 agonists causing relaxation of bronchial smooth muscles and a decrease in inflammatory mediators. Clenbuterol is rapidly absorbed with sweating, agitation, and tremors occurring at 1.6 to 6.4 μg/kg.[12,13] Doses greater than 10 μg/kg, associated with the use of illicit compounded clenbuterol, have resulted in sweating, agitation, tachycardia, arrhythmias, muscle tremors, and death.[12]Any amount of clenbuterol in horses with underlying CV disease is contraindicated. Less is known about the use of albuterol in horses but based on human studies the oral bioavailability is suspected to be low.[13,14] Most albuterol and other similar substances are administered via an inhalation device. Onset is rapid with few clinical signs observed at normal dosages.[14]

Nonsteroidal Anti-inflammatory Drugs

Many different nonsteroidal anti-inflammatory drugs (NSAIDS) have been used in horses for their analgesic, anti-inflammatory and antipyretic properties.[15] Diclofenac, dipyrone, firocoxib, flunixin meglumine, ketoprofen, and phenylbutazone (PBZ) are currently FDA approved for use in horses. Acetaminophen at 20 mg/kg and 30 mg/kg has been shown to have some success in the treatment of pain associated with lameness but the toxic dose in horses has not been established.[16] Newer NSAIDS such as firocoxib have been developed that spare cyclooygenase (COX-1) enzymes and inhibit COX-2 enzymes potentially reducing NSAID toxicity.[17] Although the use of these medications is increasing, PBZ and flunixin remain the most widely prescribed NSAIDS in horses.[15]

The margin of safety with NSAIDS is narrow and the potential for toxicosis is large, especially in neonatal foals where a longer half-life and delayed clearance play an important role.[18] In addition, individual idiosyncrasies may result in toxicosis at normal recommended dosages as will NSAID stacking. Combinations of PBZ and flunixin, PBZ and firocoxib, and PBZ and nephrotoxic drugs have all resulted in toxicosis.[15]

Gastroduodenal ulcers, right dorsal colitis (RDC), and renal papillary necrosis are documented outcomes of NSAID toxicity. These can be exacerbated by dehydration, anorexia, infectious diseases, and underlying renal or hepatic disease. Many different "toxic" dosages of PBZ are found in the literature but the most telling is that a single dose of PBZ administered IV at 13.46 mg/kg resulted in severe gastroduodenal disease including swollen and necrotic GI epithelium.[19] Right dorsal colon injury is primarily associated with chronic use of PBZ but other NSAIDS have been implicated.[20,21] Clinical signs include anorexia, diarrhea, and lethargy, with colic and fever also noted. More chronic signs include ventral edema and poorly formed feces. The earliest sign of RDC toxicosis is hypoalbuminemia followed by anemia and hypocalcemia.[20,22] Misoprostol (2–5 µg/kg PO q 6–12 hours) is the most effective treatment.[20,22] Renal papillary necrosis is reported infrequently and generally associated with dehydration, chronic renal failure, and nephrolithiasis or ureterolithiasis.[15]

Opioids

Butorphanol, buprenorphine, and meperidine are all approved for use in horses, whereas many others including fentanyl, morphine, and tramadol are not specifically approved but have widespread use. Opioid drugs are generally used therapeutically; however, their presence in a competition horse of a fentanyl patch located high in the groin area, attached to the underside of a run-down patch, or placed under a leg bandage is clearly misuse. Opioids work by binding to specific receptors located in the central nervous system (CNS), heart, GI tract, and other organs. Adverse and toxic reactions are dose related and include increased locomotion, agitation, excitation, GI stasis, respiratory depression, and death.

Most opioids are administered by injection, which allows for a rapid onset of action. A few are not. Transdermal fentanyl patches have been used successfully to provide continuous pain relief for those horses where repeated injections are not an option. The application of 2 patches (100 mcg/h each patch) for a 450 kg horse provides analgesia within 4 hours of application and lasts for 48 to 72 hours if the patches remain in place.[23] Tramadol, an oral medication, has been studied in horses but the efficacy and dosage needed to provide adequate analgesia have not been determined.[24]

Sedatives/Muscle Relaxants

Detomidine, romifidine, and xylazine are alpha-2 adrenergic agonists used alone or in combination with other drugs to produce analgesia, muscle relaxation, and sedation. Toxic effects are an extenuation of adverse events and include bradycardia, hypotension, ataxia, inability to stand, and decreased respiratory rate.[25] If xylazine is accidently given in the carotid artery, seizures and prolong duration of action occur. Death from ventricular fibrillation has been reported in one horse.[26] Yohimbine, tolazoline, and atipamezole, alpha-2 antagonists, have been used to reverse xylazine and detomidine and presumably would be reverse romifidine.[27,28]

Benzodiazepine drugs such as diazepam and alprazolam, widely used in small animal medicine, have limited use in horses, primarily due to their short half-life. The margin of safety for these drugs is wide with few toxicities reported. The most common adverse reactions include weakness, ataxia, and CNS depression.

ILLICIT MEDICATIONS AND SUPPLEMENTS
Introduction

The use of illicit medications and supplements that may be considered illicit is fraught with complications, particularly if they are compounded, or the supplements contain one or more unfamiliar herbal products. The use of either may result in a toxic reaction or a positive drug test for those horses racing under Horse Racing Integrity and Safety Authority (HISA), United States Equestrian Federation (USEF), Federation Equestre Internationale (FEI), American Quarter Horse Association (AQHA), or other breed registries.

Illicit drugs are often illegally compounded medications and associated with significant risk to the health of the horse and the potential for a positive test result. Compounded medications are not generic drugs but rather medications that are not FDA approved so there is no oversight in terms of potency, efficacy, purity, and stability. It is not unusual for compounded medications to contain less or more than specified on the label or in the case of oral suspensions become more potent as contents settle toward the bottom of the bottle.

Supplements, in particular herbal supplements, may make erroneous claims about the ingredients "not testing" but may in fact result in a positive test. As a rule, herbal supplements with capsaicin, chamomile, comfrey, devil's claw, hops, kava kava, lavender, laurel, leopard's or wolf's bane, lobelia oil, night shade, passionflower, poppy or red poppy, psilocybin, rauwolfia skullcap, valerian or valerian root, and vervain should be avoided.[29] Both valerian root and kava kava, present in many human products marketed for insomnia, have been used in horses for sedative effects and are subject to testing and penalties if present in racehorse serum or urine. In addition to capsaicin, some equine supplements contain methyl salicylate, which is similar to aspirin, and ethanol, are all illegal substances under Horseracing Integrity and Welfare Unit.

DISCUSSION
Adrenocorticotropic Hormone

Adrenocorticotropic hormone (ACTH) is a hormone released by the pituitary gland that stimulates the adrenal glands to release cortisol, corticosterone, aldosterone, and a few weak androgens. Cortisol, often referred to as the stress hormone, is an essential hormone that affects just about every body organ and plays many different roles in body function. ACTH has been used for years as an illicit drug in competition and show horses to decrease stress, suppress inflammation, and calm fractious and excitable horses.[30] It is available both as a human prescription product and through compounding pharmacies, primarily as ACTHAR gel 80 U/mL (human product) or simply as compounded ACTH gel 80 U/mL. There are no published scientific articles that provide dosing information but anecdotally 2.5 mL (200 U) is administered IM 4 to 6 hours before a competition. Repeated dosing has been associated with a rapid onset of pruritic or nonpruritic hives covering the entire body.

Anabolic Steroids

Testosterone, nandrolone, and boldenone are endogenous androgenic anabolic steroids, and trenbolone and stanozolol are the most recognized synthetic products.[31]

Commercially available forms of endogenous and synthetic products are administered to increase weight gain, improve muscle mass, and aid in the recovery of muscles weakened by long-term disease, injury, or surgery. They were once used extensively in competition horses, in particular racehorses, to increase skeletal muscle mass, enhance performance, and increase speed but improved detection by testing laboratories has led to tight regulations. This is not the end of the problem, however, as many new "designer steroids," those anabolic drugs specifically developed to avoid detection, are available on the Internet.[31] Norbolethone, tetrahydrogestrinone, and desoxymethyltestosterone (Madol or Pheraplex) are just a few offered for sale on different "steroid" websites.

Adverse and toxic reactions are common and last for weeks to months. Behavior changes including agitation, increased aggression, and dominant behavior occur most often in stallions, although mares display many of these same characteristics. In young horses, normal bone growth may be stunted resulting in short, chunky horses. Fillies and mares may seem more masculine, mount other animals, and fail to cycle normally, whereas testicular size and sperm production in stallions may be affected.[31,32]

Central Nervous System Stimulants

Cocaine is a local anesthetic drug abused by humans worldwide for the CNS effects. Both the street drug and pure cocaine are found as a powder, which can easily contaminate surfaces, hands, and horses. Based on human data, signs may occur in 5 to 10 minutes when smoke is blown into a horse's nose or within 60 minutes when applied to the mucosa.[33] Intravenous equine doses more than 0.02 mg/kg result in behavior changes and those greater than 0.04 mg/kg result in spontaneous locomotion.[34] Clinical signs include disorientation, agitation, seizures, hypertension, tachyarrhythmias, hypothermia, and rhabdomyolysis.[33]

Methylphenidate, methamphetamine, and amphetamine are all illicit drugs in horses. Methylphenidate administered IV at 0.70 mg/kg did not produce any overt clinical signs nor did an SQ injection of 0.35 mg/kg.[35] Horses dosed with 600 mg IM showed increases in the respiratory and pulse rate with CNS stimulation at 500 mg IM.[36] Methamphetamine and amphetamine are rapidly absorbed across mucous membranes reaching peak effects in 15 to 30 minutes.[37] Clinical signs of CNS stimulation, agitation, and cardiac changes are minimal at studied doses but that does not preclude them from occurring at higher doses.

Beta-2 Adrenergic Agonists

Clenbuterol, ractopamine, and zilpaterol, all beta-2 adrenergic agonists, have all been abused for their anabolic effects. The production of more muscle mass and less fat due to repartitioning effects is associated with long-term administration of clenbuterol at normal dosages or shorter term use at higher concentrations.[12] Ractopamine and zilpaterol have been used in a similar fashion.[38,39] Death is a known sequela.

Cobalt

Cobalt is an essential trace element present in feeds and many equine supplements. It is also an illicit IV medication compounded as cobalt chloride. In humans, cobalt increases red blood cell (RBC) production by stabilizing hypoxia-inducible factors. This does not occur in horses, and although the mechanism of action remains unknown, it is somehow related to an increase in performance.[40] Signs of toxicosis begin at 0.25 mg/kg and include tachycardia, arrhythmias, muscle tremors, ataxia, and anxiety with colic a common sequela.[41] In experimental cases, signs decreased about 2 hours after administration.[40]

Dermorphin

Dermorphin is a synthetic opioid derived from the skin of the South American frog (*Phyllomedusa*). As a pain reliever, the potency is stated to be 11 times greater than morphine.[42] Now highly regulated, the drug was used illicitly in racehorses to block pain, stimulate locomotor activity, and increase focus. The toxic dose is reported to be 5 mg with onset of action in 60 seconds and duration of action an hour.[42] Clinical signs include sweating, head shaking, sedation, catalepsy, increased locomotion, and colic.

Erythropoietin/Darbepoetin

Endogenous erythropoietin (EPO) is responsible for controlling the production of RBCs. Human recombinant erythropoietin (rhEPO) or darbepoetin (rhDPO), both synthetic human analogs, or illegally compounded analogs have been used illicitly to increase hematocrit and hemoglobin, maximize oxygen uptake, and increase exercise endurance time.[43,44] Both rhEPO and rhDPO are foreign products that cross react with endogenous EPO resulting in anti-rhEPO (antibodies) that inhibit erythropoiesis, resulting in severe anemia and death.[45]

Gabapentin

Gabapentin is a human prescription drug developed to mimic gamma-amino butyric acid (GABA). The mechanism of action is poorly understood but exogenous use does not affect the uptake or release of naturally occurring GABA. In some show and racehorses, gabapentin, most often associated with pain management, has been abused for its sedating effects coupled with a short detection time. Clinical signs of sedation and ataxia at higher doses occur at 1 to 2 hours after injection and resolve in about an hour.[46,47] Toxicity is low with only sedation noted at oral doses of 160 mg/kg.[46]

Growth Hormones

Growth hormone (GH) is a naturally occurring hormone needed for growth and development; recombinant GH is a synthetic drug that stimulates the release of GH. Illicit recombinant formulations purchased on the Internet or FDA-approved human or bovine recombinant products are used primarily to increase body mass and performance. The toxic effects on horses are not well understood but include injection site reactions, muscle stiffness, and adverse effects on blood glucose regulation.[48] Coadministration with anabolic steroids, beta agonists, and selective androgen receptor modulators (SARMS) increase the toxic effect.

Guanabenz

Guanabenz is an alpha-2 receptor agonist marketed for human use as antihypertensive agent. No longer available in the United States, it has been compounded as an oral or injectable product and used for sedation and to control exercise-induced pulmonary hemorrhage (EIPH). The mechanism of action is poorly understood. One theory is that EIPH is caused by pulmonary hypertension, and by lowering this risk, EIPH does not occur.[49] The anecdotal dose is 0.04 mg/kg/d either directly before a race or administered every day. Larger IV doses (0.2 mg/kg) result in rapid and profound sedation lasting up to 4 hours.[50]

Magnesium

Magnesium is an essential mineral required to maintain electrolyte balance including calcium and potassium transport, produce energy, and promote normal neuromuscular and nervous system function. It is sold in tack stores and online as an equine "calming" supplement, either alone or in combination with other substances such as thiamine, L-tryptophan, and hemp or cannabidiol. Some of these products may result in a positive test in competition horses, so again reading the label is recommended.

Intravenous magnesium sulfate has been used extensively as an illicit calming agent to "take the edge off" nervous and excitable horses before showing or racing. The mechanism of action is not understood but it may function in the CNS as an N-methyl-D aspartate receptor antagonist or in the peripheral system as a calcium channel blocker.[51] Anecdotally, 30 to 60 mL of a 50% solution is administered IV just before a competition with effects lasting anywhere from 4 to 12 hours. Laboratory detection is difficult because magnesium is an endogenous substance. Toxic effects depend on the dose administered but include excess sedation, somnolence, and hypotension.

Selective Androgen Receptor Modulators/Selective Estrogen Receptor Modulators

SARMS and selective estrogen receptor modulators (SERMS) are agonists or antagonists on androgen or estrogen receptors.[52] All SARMS are illicit medications because there are no FDA-approved products. Three SERMS are FDA approved for human use only. Several SARMS have been used for their anabolic effects in horses, with Ostarine (MK-2866) present in the postrace serum of several racehorses. In addition to performance enhancing effects, toxicosis may occur when used with other medications such as anabolic steroids, beta agonists, and GH.

DISCLOSURE

The author has no financial or commercial conflicts to disclose.

REFERENCES

1. Fletcher JR, Bertin FR, Owen H, et al. Oxytetracycline associated acute kidney injury in a neonatal foal. Equine Vet Educ 2021;33(10):e345–51.
2. Riond JL, Riviere JE, Duckett WM, et al. Cardiovascular effects and fatalities associated with intravenous administration of doxycycline to horses and ponies. Equine Vet J 1992;24(1):41–5.
3. Baird JD, Arroyo LG, Vengust M, et al. Adverse extrapyramidal effects in four horses given fluphenazine decanoate. J Am Vet Med Assoc 2006;229(1):104–10.
4. Brashier M. Fluphenazine-induced extrapyramidal side effects in a horse. Equine Clinics North Am 2006;22(1):e37–45.
5. Rodriguez-Palacios A, Quesada R, Baird J, et al. Presumptive fluphenazine-induced hepatitis and urticaria in a horse. J Vet Int Med 2007;21(2):336–9.
6. Bidwell LA, Schott HC, Derksen FJ. Reserpine toxicosis in an aged gelding. Equine Vet Educ 2007;19(7):341–3.
7. Lloyd KC, Harrison I, Tulleners E. Reserpine toxicosis in a horse. J Am Vet Med Assoc 1985;186(9):980–1.
8. Waitt Wolker LH, Veltri CA, Pearman K, et al. Pharmacokinetics of fluoxetine in horses following oral administration. J Vet Pharmacol Therapeut 2022;45(1):63–8.
9. Knych HK, Mama KR, Steffey EP, et al. Pharmacokinetics and selected pharmacodynamics of trazodone following intravenous and oral administration to horses undergoing fitness training. Am J Vet Res 2017;78(10):1182–92.
10. Davis JL, Schirmer J, Medlin E. Pharmacokinetics, pharmacodynamics and clinical use of trazodone and its active metabolite m-chlorophenylpiperazine in the horse. J Vet Pharmacol Therapeut 2018;41(3):393–401.

11. Hobbs K, Luethy D, Davis J, et al. The effects of orally administered trazodone on ambulation and recumbency in healthy horses. J Vet Int Med 2023;(Jul 25):1–8.

12. Thompson JA, Mirza MH, Barker SA, et al. Clenbuterol toxicosis in three Quarter Horse racehorses after administration of a compounded product. J Am Vet Med Assoc 2011;239(6):842–9.

13. Robinson NE. Clenbuterol and the horse. AAEP Proc 2000;26(42):229–33.

14. Derksen FJ, Olszewski MA, Robinson NE, et al. Aerosolized albuterol sulfate used as a bronchodilator in horses with recurrent airway obstruction. Am J Vet Res 1999;60(6):689–93.

15. Flood J, Stewart AJ. Non-steroidal anti-inflammatory drugs and associated toxicities in horses. Animals 2022;12(21):2939, 1-17.

16. Mercer MA, McKenzie HC, Davis JL, et al. Pharmacokinetics and safety of repeated oral dosing of acetaminophen in adult horses. Equine Vet Educ 2020; 52(1):120–5.

17. Knych HK. Nonsteroidal anti-inflammatory drug use in horses. Equine Clin North Am 2017;33(1):1–15.

18. Crisman MV, Wilcke JR, Sams RA. Pharmacokinetics of flunixin meglumine in healthy foals less than twenty-four hours old. Am J Vet Res 1996;57(12):1759–61.

19. Meschter CL, Gilbert M, Krook L, et al. The effects of phenylbutazone on the intestinal mucosa of the horse: a morphological, ultrastructural, and biochemical study. Equine Vet J 1990;22(4):255–63.

20. Davis JL. Nonsteroidal anti-inflammatory drug associated right dorsal colitis in the horse. Equine Vet Educ 2017;29(2):104–13.

21. Bishop RC, Wilkins PA, Kemper AM, et al. Effect of Firocoxib and Flunixin Meglumine on Large Colon Mural Thickness of Healthy Horses. J Equine Vet Sci 2023; 126:104562, 1-6.

22. Cohen ND. Right dorsal colitis. Equine Vet Educ 2002;14(4):212–9.

23. Matthews NS, Carroll GL. Review of equine analgesics and pain management. Orlando, Florida: Proceedings of the Annual Convention of the American association of equine Practitioners; 2007. p. 240–4.

24. Knych HK, Corado CR, McKemie DS, et al. Pharmacokinetics and pharmacodynamics of tramadol in horses following oral administration. J Vet Pharmacol Therapeut 2013;36(4):389–98.

25. Wagner AE, Muir WW, Hinchcliff KW. Cardiovascular effects of xylazine and detomidine in horses. Am J Vet Res 1981;52(5):651–7.

26. Fuentes VO. Sudden death in a stallion after xylazine medication. Vet Rec 1978; 102(5):106.

27. Kollias-Baker CA, Court MH, Williams LL. Influence of yohimbine and tolazoline on the cardiovascular, respiratory, and sedative effects of xylazine in the horse. J Vet Pharmacol Therapeut 1993;16(3):350–8.

28. Ramseyer B, Schmucker N, Schatzmann U, et al. Antagonism of detomidine sedation with atipamezole in horses. J Vet Anesth 1998;(1):47–51.

29. Dasgupta A. Toxic herbals and plants in the United States. In: Toxicology cases for the clinical and forensic laboratory. London: Academic Press; 2020. p. 359–68.

30. Caloni F, Spotti M, Villa R, et al. Hydrocortisone levels in the urine and blood of horses treated with ACTH. Equine Vet J 1999;31(4):273–6.

31. Dirikolu L, Lehner AF. A review of current chemistry, pharmacology, and regulation of endogenous anabolic steroids testosterone, boldenone, and nandrolone in horses. J Vet Pharmacol Therapeut 2023;46(4):201–17.

32. Soma LR, Udoh CE, Guan F, et al. Pharmacokinetics of boldenone and stanozolol and the results of quantification of anabolic and androgenic steroids in racehorses and nonrace horses. J Vet Pharmacol Therapeut 2007;30(2):101–8.
33. Cole C. Cocaine. In: Hovda LR, Benson D, Poppenga RS, editors. Blackwell's five-minute veterinary Consult clinical Companion: equine toxicology. New Jersey: Wiley; 2022. p. 41–4.
34. Queiroz-Neto A, Zamur G, Lacerda-Neto JC, et al. Determination of the highest no-effect dose (HNED) and of the elimination pattern for cocaine in horses. J Appl Toxicon 2002;22(2):117–21.
35. Shults T, Kownacki AA, Woods WE, et al. Pharmacokinetics and behavioral effects of methylphenidate in Thoroughbred horses. Am J Vet Res 1981;42(5): 722–6.
36. Gabriel KL, Henderson B, Smith WF. Studies on the physiologic effects of methylphenidate in thoroughbred horses. J Am Vet Med Assoc 1963;142:875–7.
37. Knych HK, Arthur RM, Kanarr KL, et al. Detection, pharmacokinetics, and selected pharmacodynamic effects of methamphetamine following a single transmucosal and intravenous administration to exercised Thoroughbred horses. Drug Test Anal 2019;11(9):1431–43.
38. Lehner AF, Hughes CG, Harkins JD, et al. Detection and confirmation of ractopamine and its metabolites in horse urine after Paylean® administration. J Anal Toxicol 2004;28(4):226–37.
39. Wagner SA, Mostrom MS, Hammer CJ, et al. Adverse effects of zilpaterol administration in horses: three cases. J Eq Vet Sci 2008;28(4):238–43.
40. Knych HK, Arthur RM, Mitchell MM, et al. Pharmacokinetics and selected pharmacodynamics of cobalt following a single intravenous administration to horses. Drug Test Anal 2015;7(7):619–25.
41. Burns TA, Dembek KA, Kamr A, et al. Effect of intravenous administration of cobalt chloride to horses on clinical and hemodynamic variables. J Vet Int Med 2018;32(1):441–9.
42. Robinson MA, Guan F, McDonnell S, et al. Pharmacokinetics and pharmacodynamics of dermorphin in the horse. J Vet Pharmacol Therapeut 2015;38(4):321–9.
43. McKeever KH, Agans JM, Geiser S, et al. Low dose exogenous erythropoietin elicits an ergogenic effect in standardbred horses. Equine Vet J 2006;38(S36): 233–8.
44. Guan F, Uboh CE, Soma LR, et al. LC– MS/MS method for confirmation of recombinant human erythropoietin and darbepoetin α in equine plasma. Anal Chem 2007;79(12):4627–35.
45. Piercy RJ, Swardson CJ, Hinchcliff KW. Erythroid hypoplasia and anemia following administration of recombinant human erythropoietin to two horses. J Am Vet Med Assoc 1998;212(2):244–7.
46. Terry RL, McDonnell SM, Van Eps AW, et al. Pharmacokinetic profile and behavioral effects of gabapentin in the horse. J Vet Pharmacol Therapeut 2010;33(5): 485–94.
47. Gold JR, Grubb TL, Green S, et al. Plasma disposition of gabapentin after the intragastric administration of escalating doses to adult horses. J Vet Int Med 2020; 34(2):933–40.
48. Moeller BC. Growth Hormone and Secretagogues. In: Hovda LR, Benson D, Poppenga RS, editors. Blackwell's five-minute veterinary Consult clinical Companion: equine toxicology. New Jersey: Wiley; 2022. p. 49052.
49. Harkins JD, Dirikolu L, Lehner AF, et al. The detection and biotransformation of guanabenz in horses: a preliminary report. Vet Therp 2003;4(2):197–209.

50. Lehner A, Dirikolu L, Tobin T. Guanabenz in the horse–A preliminary report on clinical effects and comparison to clonidine and other alpha-2 adrenergic agonists. Pferdeheilkunde 2022;38(6):554–65.
51. Schumacher SA, Toribio RE, Scansen B, et al. Pharmacokinetics of magnesium and its effects on clinical variables following experimentally induced hypermagnesemia. J Vet Pharmacol Therapeut 2020;43(6):577–90.
52. Hansson A, Knych H, Stanley S, et al. Characterization of equine urinary metabolites of selective androgen receptor modulators (SARMs) S1, S4 and S22 for doping control purposes. Drug Test Anal 2015;7(8):673–83.

Ionophores

Scott A. Fritz, DVM[a],*, Jeffery O. Hall, DVM, PhD[b]

KEYWORDS

- Ionophores • Horse • Heart failure • Toxicity • Monensin

KEY POINTS

- Horses are extremely sensitive to the toxic effects of ionophores.
- Ionophores disrupt ion gradients that eventually result in cell death.
- Myocardial damage is the most significant effect in horses.
- Poisoning can occur via exposure to feeds or supplements meant for other species or inadvertent inclusion of ionophores in horse feeds.
- There is no antidote for ionophore toxicosis.

INTRODUCTION

Ionophores are polyether carboxylic antibiotics used as feed additives in many species for their anticoccidial activity, as well as for their ability to increase feed efficiency and rate of gain in ruminants. Specific ionophores commonly used today include laidlomycin propionate, lasalocid, maduramicin, monensin, narasin, and salinomycin. The widespread use of these compounds in animal feeds is a risk factor for exposure of non-target species. Cases of toxicosis involving these compounds typically result from misformulations of feed concentrations or exposure of non-target species to dietary concentrations that are safe for the intended species. Field cases have been reported in horses, cattle, sheep, turkeys, pigs, dogs, cats, rabbits, white-tailed deer, guinea fowls, ostriches, and chickens.[1] Horses are uniquely sensitive to these compounds and exposure should be avoided.

As the name suggests, ionophores are capable of moving ions across biological membranes and down concentration gradients. These biological membranes include both cellular and organelle membranes. Cells and organelles have energy-driven membrane pumps that maintain ion gradients. The capability of the cell or organelle to maintain ion gradients is eventually exceeded in cases of ionophore toxicosis which results in damage at the cellular and organelle level. The organelle that suffers the

[a] Department of Anatomy and Physiology, Kansas State University College of Veterinary Medicine, 1620 Denison Avenue, 228 Coles Hall, Manhattan, KS 66506, USA; [b] Cattle Technical Services, Huvepharma Inc., 525 Westpark Dr, Suite 230, Peachtree City, GA 30269, USA
* Corresponding author. 1620 Denison Avenue, 228 Coles Hall, Manhattan, KS 66506.
E-mail address: scottfritz@vet.k-state.edu

most damage following ingestion of a toxic dose of an ionophore is the mitochondria. Mitochondrial damage results in the loss of ATP production, which is used to drive the ion pumps that normally maintain ion gradients across membranes. This compounds the effects at the cellular level and eventually results in death of the cell.

There is significant interspecies variability in the tissue effects of the different ionophores. In horses, cardiac muscle is the primary site of damage, though some damage also can occur to the skeletal muscle, neurologic tissue, liver, and kidney. There is also intraspecies variability in how individual animals respond to a given dose, making prognostic recommendations for a single patient difficult for practitioners. The clinical presentation of toxicosis to the various ionophore compounds in horses is similar and mainly revolves around cardiac effects. Exposed animals can succumb to ionophore exposure acutely, and those that survive the initial insult may succumb to compromised cardiac function months after the exposure. While some animals can have a long-term functional life as breeding animals, exercise and performance ability deficits should be expected. The stresses of breeding and foaling could also exacerbate ionophore-induced cardiac damage. Toxic exposures to a large group of animals typically result in multiple manifestations of effects over time.

Diagnosis of ionophore toxicosis is ideally accomplished with physical examination, clinical pathologic data, specialized heart evaluation, and in death-loss events, with gross and histologic lesions after necropsy. The diagnosis can be supported by quantification of the offending compound in feeds and occasionally in tissues. Feed testing is inherently challenging due to the potential delay from consumption to clinical presentation, variable distribution of the offending compound in a given quantity of feed, and the potential for multiple compounds being present while only analyzing for one specifically.

DISCUSSION

Ionophores are widely used feed additives in diets for food-producing animals, and the proximity of horses to many of these operations makes inadvertent exposure a relatively common occurrence. The toxic dose of a given ionophore varies with the compound as well as the individual animal exposed. Lethal doses of the various ionophore compounds are presented in **Table 1**. Given that the reported LD_{50}s are doses that result in a lethality of 50%, lower doses can also be lethal, and minimum toxic doses in larger groups of horses have not been established for the ionophores. Ionophores have a relatively steep toxic response curve, and case evaluations have found that

Table 1
Oral toxicity of various ionophores for horses[2]

Ionophore	LD_{50} (mg/kg)	Other	References
Lasalocid	21.5		Hanson et al,[3] 1981
Monensin	2–3		Todd et al,[4] 1984
Narasin		Lethal dose not reported	
Salinomycin	0.6		Van et al,[5] 1985
Laidlomycin propionate		Lethal at 6.6 mg/kg 1 day Lethal at 2.86 mg/kg for 5 d	Hall et al,[6] 1996
Maduramycin		Lethal dose not reported	

From: **Hall JO**: Toxic Feed Constituents in the Horse. W.B. Saunders Company. Vet Clin North Am Equine Pract 17(3): 479-489, 2001.

one should not expect to see adverse effects at doses of less than 10% of the reported LD_{50}. Thus, very low amounts can result in nontoxic exposures.

It is important to recognize that a single overdose can result in clinical signs and death. Often the first clinical sign observed is anorexia,[6-8] but this can occur after a lethal dose has already been ingested. Multiple dosing studies in multiple species have shown repeat exposures of lower doses can also cause death,[9] although the anorexia observed in field cases may prevent this occurrence in natural exposures.

Clinical Signs

The clinical progression of toxicosis typically develops within a couple of hours of exposure. The clinical syndrome is characterized by anorexia, weakness/ataxia, tremors, exaggerated gait, reluctance to move, tachycardia, jugular pulse, dyspnea, sweating, recumbency, and death.[1,7,8,10-12] Affected animals may continue to eat hay. Death can occur in horses within 24 hours of exposure or can be delayed for several days to weeks depending upon the compound, dose, and individual susceptibility of the animal. Multiple case reports have detailed the long-term effects of ionophore toxicosis.[8,10,13,14] While these reports detailed some horses dying initially, this progressed to multiple other horses from the same place developing varying signs of poor performance, exercise intolerance, ataxia, weakness, muscle atrophy, and tachycardia over the course of several months.

Minimum Database

Clinicopathologic abnormalities in horses are generally associated with muscle and liver damage. These changes are variable between horses and include elevations in creatine phosphokinase, lactate dehydrogenase, aspartate aminotransferase, alkaline phosphatase, blood urea nitrogen glucose, osmolality, hematocrit, and phosphorous. Increased urine volume with decreased osmolality was reported in multiple case reports, as well as decreased serum calcium and potassium. The variability of these alterations and the timing of occurrence between individual horses make their usefulness in monitoring clinical patients more difficult but can be used to support a diagnosis. As development of clinicopathologic changes can be acute or delayed, repeated testing (daily or every other day over a 10–14-day period) of each exposed animal would be necessary to have some certainty of identifying adverse effects in individual animals.

Electrocardiogram tracings have been reported in field exposures and dosing studies using monensin and salinomycin.[6,14] Abnormalities, such as increased S-wave amplitude, absent P-wave, atrial fibrillation, intermittent premature ventricular contractions, ventricular tachycardia, and atrioventricular block among others, were identified occasionally, though not consistently, and the abnormalities themselves were not always repeatable. The variability limits electrocardiogram's usefulness in clinical evaluations. Echocardiography identification of altered fractional shortening of the ventricular myocardium has also been reported in ionophore-poisoned horses.

Cardiac troponin I (cTnI) is a sensitive biomarker of myocardial injury in humans[15] and has been used in animals.[16] A dosing study utilized cTnI analysis following monensin administration to horses and determined cTnI can be used to separate those with myocardial damage from those without, especially in group exposures.[7] The severity of cTnI elevation could provide some prognostic data.[7] With the increasing availability of animal-side cTnI assays (i-STAT, Abbott, Abbott Park, IL, USA), cTnI is likely the most practical method to determine the severity of damage and the potential for return to use for many horses in cases of ionophore toxicosis. As with the other clinicopathologic parameters, repeated testing over a 10 to 14-day period may be needed to catch those animals that have a more delayed cardiotoxic effect.

Treatment

There is no specific antidote for ionophore toxicosis. Clinical management of exposed horses depends upon the dose consumed and the severity of the disease. Activated charcoal given orally within a couple of hours of ingestion should limit some absorption. Vitamin E and selenium supplementation has shown some benefit when given prior to an ionophore overdose in other species;[17] however, their efficacy once animals develop clinical signs is questionable. Stall rest is imperative in clinical animals as exercise can result in acute death.

Postmortem

Abnormalities observed during gross necropsy evaluation are typically directly or indirectly associated with the effects on the myocardium. Direct observations include pale streaks in the myocardium, friability of the myocardium, generalized pallor, and endocardial or epicardial hemorrhage.[1,7,8,12] Observations indirectly related to myocardial damage include bicavitary effusion, pulmonary congestion and edema, hyperemic kidneys, urinary bladder distention, hepatic congestion with lobular pattern, and edema of multiple tissues.[1,7,8]

Microscopic lesions are typically relegated to the myocardium.[1,7,8] Myocardial degeneration and necrosis are the hallmark lesions of intoxication, but the time of evaluation in relation to the exposure can affect the lesions observed. Some animals can die quickly enough that death precedes histologic lesion formation, whereas others live long enough to develop visible histologic lesions. In delayed cases, the histologic lesions are more chronic in nature, with significant fibrosis and varying degrees of mineralization replacing the necrotic areas. Dosing studies have reported variable renal and hepatic lesions as well, including vacuolar hepatopathy, centrilobular hepatocyte degeneration and necrosis, tubular nephritis, and renal tubular necrosis with myoglobin casts.[6] Some of the hepatic and renal lesions are likely a secondary consequence of heart failure and heart muscle damage.

Feed Testing

Many diagnostic laboratories offer feed testing for monensin and the other ionophores. It is important to recognize that feed mills producing feed for multiple species can have many different ionophores in use. Failure to adequately flush the manufacturing or distribution equipment can result in multiple ionophores being present in any given feed. The effects of multiple ionophore compounds can be expected to be synergistic and if only one is quantified, a true representation of the potential toxic exposure may be missed. Testing feed can be frustrating in that most feeds are not completely homogenous. There may be "hot spots" in any bulk-produced feed that can be responsible for a toxic exposure to 1 or more animals of a particular group. Analyzing a small subsample of a larger bulk sample can result in an inadequate interpretation of the exposure. The best recommendation is to take multiple "grab samples" from several different areas or bags, combine and mix those, and then submit a sample of the mixed grab samples for analysis. Results can then be back calculated to form an estimate of the dosage consumed. Further testing of multiple individual grab samples or samples from multiple bags can aid in determining the variability and aid in the evaluation of maximal potential exposure. Exposure estimation is further compounded when multiple animals are fed as a group as individual intake will vary.

Tissue Analysis

Tissue testing is available at some laboratories for specific ionophores. Ionophores are rapidly absorbed and metabolized and are not stored in tissues for prolonged periods of time making the development of tissue reference ranges impractical. One report detailed the analysis of tissue concentrations in multiple field cases, and ultimately tissue concentrations did not correlate with clinical disease or severity of lesions.[11] The heart had the highest concentration of drug of the analyzed tissues and is likely the best specimen for analytical testing. Tissue concentrations can be used to identify exposure and support a diagnosis when combined with clinical disease, gross lesions, and histologic lesions; however, tissue concentrations alone are not sufficient to reach a diagnosis.

In many field cases of ionophore intoxication, there is a distribution of effects in exposed animals. Some animals may die acutely, while other animals may have less severe clinical signs that lead to death several weeks later. Other exposed animals may survive. This distribution is a function of many factors including nonhomogeneity of mixed feeds, individual intake/dosage, and individual susceptibility.

SUMMARY

Horses are extremely sensitive to ionophores, a group of antibiotic compounds that are widely used in production animal operations. Their widespread use makes mistakes in formulations for target species and exposure of non-target species relatively common. Ionophores act by transporting ions across lipid membranes and can disturb ion gradients resulting in decreased energy production and cell death. The myocardium is the primary target of ionophores in horses, and the death of cardiomyocytes is responsible for the clinical syndrome appreciated after exposure. It should follow that the degree of collective damage to individual cells is related to the clinical outcome. Clinical signs initially reflect some gastrointestinal disturbance (anorexia, diarrhea, colic) and progress to evidence of cardiac compromise (exercise intolerance, reluctance to move, jugular pulse, respiratory distress). Morbidity and mortality can be relatively high in horses fed as a group but will be related to the dose received. Animals can die within 24 hours, and some may live weeks to months depending on the severity of damage to the heart. Diagnosis is typically based on histologic evaluation of the heart, as well as feed and potentially tissue testing for ionophore compounds. There is no antidote for ionophore poisoning, and treatment is largely supportive. Some affected animals may be able to recover enough to perform in breeding programs, but affected sport horses should not be expected to make a complete recovery for competitions following clinical disease.

CLINICS CARE POINTS

- Horses are more sensitive to ionophores than other species where ionophores are utilized.
- Horses experience myocardial damage after ingestion of a toxic dose.
- Clinical signs are related to cardiac compromise.
- Cardiac troponins can be utilized to identify diseased animals and potentially provide some prognostic indicators based upon the severity of the elevation.
- There is no specific antidote for ionophore toxicosis.
- Supportive care and stall rest are the currently recommended practices.
- Recovered animals will likely experience a long-term reduction in physical performance.

- Diagnosis is best accomplished with histopathology and chemical detection of ionophores in feed.

DISCLOSURE

The authors have no disclosures to make.

REFERENCES

1. Hall JO. Feed-Associated Toxicants: Ionophores. In: Plumlee K, editor. Clinical veterinary toxicology. St. Louis, MO: Mosby; 2004. p. 120–7.
2. Hall JO. Toxic feed constituents in the horse. Vet Clin N Am Equine Pract 2001;17: 479–89, vii.
3. Hanson LJ, Eisenbeis HG, Givens SV. Toxic effects of lasalocid in horses. Am J Vet Res 1981;42:456–61.
4. Todd G, Novilla M, Howard L. Comparative toxicology of monensin sodium in laboratory animals. J Anim Sci 1984;58:1512–7.
5. Van Amstel S, Guthrie A. Salinomycin poisoning in horses: case report. USA: Proceedings of the annual convention of the American Association of Equine Practitioners; 1985.
6. Hall JO. Mechanisms of ionophore toxicoses: Laidlomycin propionate toxicosis in the horse, Laidlomycin propionate, Laidlomycin, and monensin in muscle cell cultures. University of Illinois; 1996.
7. Divers TJ, Kraus MS, Jesty SA, et al. Clinical findings and serum cardiac troponin I concentrations in horses after intragastric administration of sodium monensin. J Vet Diagn Invest 2009;21:338–43.
8. Decloedt A, Verheyen T, De Clercq D, et al. Acute and long-term cardiomyopathy and delayed neurotoxicity after accidental lasalocid poisoning in horses. J Vet Intern Med 2012;26:1005–11.
9. Potter EL, VanDuyn RL, Cooley CO. Monensin toxicity in cattle. J Anim Sci 1984; 58:1499–511.
10. Aleman M, Magdesian KG, Peterson TS, et al. Salinomycin toxicosis in horses. J Am Vet Med Assoc 2007;230:1822–6.
11. Bautista AC, Tahara J, Mete A, et al. Diagnostic value of tissue monensin concentrations in horses following toxicosis. J Vet Diagn Invest 2014;26:423–7.
12. Peek SF, Marques FD, Morgan J, et al. Atypical Acute Monensin Toxicosis and Delayed Cardiomyopathy in Belgian Draft Horses. J Vet Intern Med 2004;18:761–4.
13. Muylle E, Vandenhende C, Oyaert W, et al. Delayed monensin sodium toxicity in horses. Equine Vet J 1981;13:107–8.
14. Gy C, Leclere M, Bélanger MC, et al. Acute, subacute and chronic sequelae of horses accidently exposed to monensin-contaminated feed. Equine Vet J 2020;52:848–56.
15. Hjortshøj S, Dethlefsen C, Kristensen SR, et al. Improved assay of cardiac troponin I is more sensitive than other assays of necrosis markers. Scand J Clin Lab Investig 2008;68:130–3.
16. O'Brien PJ. Cardiac troponin is the most effective translational safety biomarker for myocardial injury in cardiotoxicity. Toxicology 2008;245:206–18.
17. Van Vleet JF, Amstutz HE, Weirich WE, et al. Acute monensin toxicosis in swine: effect of graded doses of monensin and protection of swine by pretreatment with selenium-vitamin E. Am J Vet Res 1983;44:1460–8.

Industrial and Agricultural Toxicants

Scott Radke, DVM, MS*, Emily Finley, DVM

KEYWORDS

- Agricultural • Equine • Industrial • Toxins

KEY POINTS

- There is a wide variety of agricultural and industrial compounds that may be encountered by equids, including fertilizers, gases, metals, and pesticides.
- Although several agricultural and industrial compounds are considered to be toxic, poisonings in equids may not be common for all compounds.
- Information regarding toxicities may need to be extrapolated from other species because few data are available for many compounds in regards to their effects on equids.

INTRODUCTION

There are numerous agricultural and industrial chemicals that are widely used in a variety of ways. These compounds are available in many different formulations and physical states. Some have little to no toxic potential, whereas others can have devastating consequences following consumption or direct exposure. Much like the vast quantity of agents that horses and other animals may be exposed to, there is an equal, if not greater, number of inquiries made pertaining to these compounds regarding equine health. The focus of this article is to provide information about several common toxic agents found within agriculture and industry that horses may encounter.

ANHYDROUS AMMONIA

Anhydrous ammonia (AA) is often used as a nitrogen fertilizer applied to soil for both row and cover crops.[1] It appears as a white plume during use or following leaks because of both its highly pressurized nature in specialized tanks and contact with moisture.[2] Although poisonings associated with AA in equine have not been reported extensively within the literature, its widespread use in agricultural settings, and proximity of application and storage sites to horses, presents risk of exposure.[2,3] There is a single report of a horse being affected through chronic exposure following an incident with a broken pipeline.[2] Potential sources of exposure could include equipment

Iowa State University College of Veterinary Medicine, Veterinary Diagnostic and Production Animal Medicine, 1850 Christensen Drive, Ames, IA 50011, USA
* Corresponding author.
E-mail address: slradke@iastate.edu

malfunctions or damage including broken valves, tank leaks, and the improper storage of such tanks near animals. Broken equipment may also be the result of attempted AA theft for methamphetamine production.[3] Improper application in windy conditions can also result in exposure.[2] Producers and veterinarians should also be aware that AA exposure presents a significant human health concern.[4]

AA, when released, will seek out any source of water including biological tissues and fluids. The high water content within mucus membranes makes these tissues particularly susceptible to AA. Upon contacting water, AA is transformed into the alkali ammonium hydroxide (NH_4OH). NH_4OH is extremely caustic, resulting in severe burns.[1,5] The eyes, oral cavity, and respiratory tract are particularly susceptible and rapidly develop lesions. Onset of clinical signs is immediate. Ocular irritation, indicated by increased lacrimation, and coughing are often observed.[2] Apnea can develop due to damaged airways, rapidly resulting in death. Sloughing of the muzzle and respiratory tract epithelium and corneal damage are expected. Significant damage to the eyes may leave animals blind.[3] Following chronic exposure and persistent ocular irritation, one equine exposed to AA was thought to then be predisposed to increased incidence of ocular carcinomas.[2] The prognosis for surviving animals is poor because survivors are susceptible to secondary infections due to the loss of respiratory epithelium. Initial treatment is irrigation of the eyes and other exposed areas. Follow-up treatment is supportive at best and requires an intensive antibiotic regimen.[1,3]

ETHYLENE GLYCOL

Ethylene glycol (EG) is found in various antifreeze products, and intoxications are often referred to as "antifreeze poisoning."[6] However, some antifreeze products contain propylene glycol (PG) rather than EG.[7] Although EG poisonings in horses are not widely reported within the literature, they do occur.[8] Sources of EG intoxication in equines include inadvertent exposure to EG-containing antifreeze for example, spills, improper storage, and improperly discarded fluids following radiator flushes and change of vehicle fluids.[8,9] Malicious poisonings with EG in horses, although uncommon in peer-reviewed literature, have been reported in media.

Following ingestion, EG is rapidly metabolized by alcohol dehydrogenase to glycoaldehyde within the liver.[10] Glycoaldehyde is further metabolized into first glycolic acid and then glycoxylic acid. Oxalic acid, the metabolic product of glyoxylic acid, combines with calcium resulting in the formation of calcium oxalate crystals. These crystals directly damage renal tubular epithelium resulting in renal failure. Although not commonly observed or reported, deposition of crystals may also occur within the vasculature of the brain.[6,10,11]

Signs associated with early EG poisoning are akin to those of PG (see later discussion).[12,13] Onset of clinical signs is likely to occur within 8 hours following ingestion. Horses may exhibit ataxia, sweating, agitation, and become neurologically depressed. Affected individuals may also become both hypothermic and tachycardic. Bloodwork is likely to reveal acidosis with an increased anion gap and increased sorbitol dehydrogenase.[8] Animals may also become hypokalemic, hypochloremic, and hyperglycemic. Practitioners should be aware that these findings may also be observed if the horse is treated for EG intoxication with ethanol.

Suspected EG poisoning can be confirmed through direct detection of the compound respectively.[11] Detection of EG in urine can be performed either with a bench side test kit or through gas chromatography flame ionization detector (GC-FID).[8] EG can be detected in gastrointestinal (GI) content through gas chromatography-mass spectrometry (GC-MS).[9] The bench top test, although relatively quick, is subjective in nature and may provide both false positives and negatives. The GC-MS approach is specific and quantitative but is more time consuming and requires specialized equipment.[11] Some GC-FID methods also have the benefit of detecting glycolic acid, which is useful if EG has been completely metabolized or is no longer present.[8] Observation of calcium crystals in urine may be of little diagnostic value because the excretion of calcium carbonate and calcium oxalate dihydrate crystals occurs normally in equines. Postmortem submission of liver and kidney may also be used to detect the compounds in question as well as provide microscopic evidence of poisoning in renal tissue.[9]

Treatment of EG poisoning must be performed quickly with the goal of inhibiting its metabolism. Treatment can be achieved through the intravenous administration of fluids and diluted ethanol. An initial 10-L bolus of lactated ringers solution (LRS) followed by continuous intravenous administration of LRS at a dosage of 140 mL/kg/d along with ethanol (95%) at 20% in normal saline at a dose of 2.5 mL/kg was reported to successfully treat a horse that had ingested EG-based antifreeze that had been in a bucket of water.[8] The 20% solution of ethanol and saline was administered every 4 hours and titrated as treatment progressed. To prevent ethanol poisoning during treatment, blood ethanol content should be monitored closely and dosage adjusted accordingly. Individuals with a blood ethanol concentration of 126.57 mmol/L are likely to become severely depressed and unresponsive to stimuli. Recovery may take several days.

FERTILIZERS

Fertilizers are compounds applied to soils to encourage plant growth. These compounds are widely used in agricultural settings, particularly for crops. The most common types of fertilizers are nitrate-based, urea-based, or phosphate-based.[14,15] Although poisonings associated with fertilizers, particularly nitrate and urea-based forms, are common in ruminants, poisonings in horses are rare.[14,16] As such, there are less data regarding fertilizer poisoning in the literature with the exception of a single case involving a nitrate-based compound.[17] Large quantities of urea administered to ponies resulted in morbidity and mortality.[18] The GI physiology of horses minimizes the effects of urea ingestion. The most likely source of fertilizer poisoning in equines is direct ingestion of highly concentrated material from recent application to forages, storage containers, misformulated feed, or contaminated water.[17,18]

Fertilizers may act through a variety of mechanisms depending on the type in question. In horses, direct irritation of the GI tract is the most common expectation for all fertilizers.[14] Nitrate-based forms may result in the formation of methemoglobin resulting in respiratory distress and anoxia.[17] Urea-based products exert their toxic effects following metabolism to ammonia leading to neurologic deficits.[18] However, both nitrate and urea must first be metabolized to their toxic metabolites, nitrite and ammonia, respectively. These metabolic processes take place within the cecum but to a much lesser extent than in the rumen of a ruminant. Due to the limited metabolic capacity of these 2 compounds, the chances of achieving concentrations high enough to cause respiratory and neurologic complications is minimal but can happen with high concentrations.[17,18]

Ataxia, incoordination, head pressing, tremors, and seizures can occur with both nitrate-based and urea-based fertilizers.[17,18] Nitrate intoxication can also cause respiratory distress and cyanotic mucous membranes.[17] GI inflammation may be the only lesion observed on postmortem evaluation. An ammonia odor within the GI tract may be present with urea-associated cases, whereas chocolate-colored blood may be present in cases of nitrate poisoning.[17,18] Diagnosis of fertilizer poisoning relies heavily on history of exposure and type of product. Forage and suspect material should be submitted for analysis at minimum. Postmortem ocular fluid and cecal content should be collected for analysis of either nitrate or ammonia. Samples should be collected as soon as possible, sealed, and frozen. Serum is the preferred antemortem sample for nitrate and ammonia.[16] Treatment is supportive, and prognosis is generally good unless large quantities of concentrate are consumed.[14,15]

METALS
Arsenic

Arsenic (As) is a naturally occurring element in most soils in minute concentrations. Common sources include desiccants, wood preservatives, select herbicides, and old insecticides.[19] However, the use of arsenicals within feeds is no longer practiced. Chronic As intoxication is uncommon in equids because As is efficiently excreted from the body. Acute intoxications are possible. Severe GI and renal damages are associated with this metal.[20]

Horses experiencing As intoxication may salivate heavily, tremble, or exhibit weakness. Tachycardia and hyperemic mucus membranes may be observed. Due to the effects on the GI tract, afflicted individuals are likely to experience severe colic with dark green to black diarrhea.[20] Diagnosis relies on the combination of the aforementioned observed clinical signs, history of exposure, lesions, and detection of As within the urine (>10 mg/L) or within liver or kidney (>7 and 10 mg/kg, respectively).[20,21] Normal levels in the liver and kidney should be less than 0.5 ppm.[21] Death often occurs within 24 hours of a fatal dose. Animals that survive to 48 hours postingestion or beyond may recover. Treatment primarily relies on intensive fluid therapy paired with intravenous sodium thiosulfate to bind unabsorbed As. Dimercaprol in horses may also be considered to be of additional benefit, if available. Flunixin meglumine may be used to treat abdominal pain. Supportive care to address GI and renal damage is usually warranted.[20,22]

Iron

Iron (Fe) is an essential nutrient required for numerous physiologic processes but can be detrimental in excess. Water and diet serve as the primary sources of Fe in horses. Forage sources, such as alfalfa, have been reported to possess concentrations of greater than 700 mg/kg.[19] Forage originating from poor soils may have as little as 40 mg/kg Fe. Fe intoxications are not a common occurrence in equine but there have been some reported cases through means of excessive supplementation. Examples of such occurrences include injectable products in racing and endurance industries. Young foals are particularly susceptible to oral oversupplementation due to an increased absorptive capacity of the GI tract. High Fe in the equine diet is frequently the result of soil contamination.[23]

Excessive Fe in the diet may result in direct GI damage due to its corrosive nature. This may lead to hepatopathy, which can progress to multiple organ failure in very extreme cases. Coagulopathies may occur secondary to liver damage. A thoroughbred with Fe toxicosis experienced excessive bleeding after diagnostic procedures as well as visible icterus on presentation.[24] Chronic Fe toxicosis can affect the liver, heart, and pancreatic beta cells primarily because it is hypothesized that excessive intracellular Fe has detrimental effects to the mitochondria of cells. The extent of tissue damage from excess Fe absorption depends heavily on the antioxidant status of the animal.[25] Animals are much more tolerant of high dietary Fe exposure compared to high-Fe water.[19]

Equine serum Fe concentrations greater than 400 μg/dL indicate acute Fe intoxication with peak levels occurring within 4 hours after exposure. Although more difficult to obtain ante mortem, the liver is a more stable indicator of Fe status than serum, and biopsies are the best diagnostic option. Hepatic Fe concentrations greater than 600 mg/kg wet weight indicate intoxication. Treatment could include chelation with deferoxamine because it has been implemented successfully in small animals. Veterinarians and owners should be aware that successful use of this chelator results in red/brown urine as Fe is excreted. High dietary calcium concentrations, as well as high phytate diets, seem to be beneficial in reducing Fe toxicity potential. Supplemental vitamin E can reduce detrimental effects of high-Fe intake.[19,24]

Lead

Much like As, lead (Pb) is found in the environment via soils and water naturally in small concentrations. However, Pb is a prominent toxicant in veterinary medicine. Acute Pb poisoning in horses can occur from ingestion of Pb batteries, Pb-based paint and paint chips from buildings built before 1960, ashes or mortar from these old buildings, crankcase oil, and forages grown in soil contaminated by these materials. Pb toxicosis in horses is much less common than in cattle and dogs but it still happens.[26,27]

Pb is primarily absorbed within the GI tract because the acidic environment of the stomach and proximal duodenum provide an environment that is conducive for absorption. Ultimately, only about 10% of ingested Pb is absorbed and available to the equine body. Chronic exposure to small amounts of Pb over time may result in deposition into bones, which can result in anemia and peripheral neuropathy in the horse. Acute Pb toxicosis results in more dramatic clinical complications with detrimental effects to the central nervous system (CNS). Intoxicated horses may exhibit muscle fasciculations, hyperesthesia, severe neurologic symptoms such as convulsions, laryngeal hemiplegia, and concurrent "roaring" possibly inducing aspiration pneumonia, colic, and GI upset.[26,28] Weight loss maybe witnessed in the animal along with muscle fasciculations and general discomfort clinically presenting very similarly to equine degenerative lower motor neuron disease.[27] Diagnosis of acute poisoning can be made on correlation of clinical signs and either whole blood Pb concentrations of greater than 0.6 mg/kg or liver and kidney concentrations greater than 10 and 20 mg/kg wet weight, respectively.[21]

Treatment strategies focus on maximizing elimination via urination and chelation. Calcium disodium sodium calcium edetate is calcium disodium EDTA (Ca-EDTA) increases Pb excretion from the blood and soft tissue but not bone. This treatment can be administered at 75 mg/kg, ideally divided into 3 separate treatments per day and made into a 6.6% solution of Ca-EDTA with normal saline or 5% dextrose. Four days of treatment followed by two days rest then 4 days of treatment was utilized.[27] Administration of intravenous (IV) fluids aids with the excretion of Pb and rehydration. Blood Pb concentration can be checked within 2 weeks of last chelation treatment, and if levels are greater than 0.35 ppm, the treatment should be repeated.

Zinc

Zinc (Zn) is an essential trace mineral but can be harmful in excess. Very few Zn intoxications have been reported in equines. Individuals in such cases exhibited lameness and failed to thrive. Osteochondrosis was noted in foals.[29] Nutritional Zn has a direct impact on copper metabolism in foals.[30] Zn status can be evaluated through either serum or liver. Practitioners should be aware that certain blood collection tubes (tiger-striped serum separators) can artificially increase Zn serum levels within a sample as the stopper and lubricant contain Zn. If red top tubes must be used, storage in an upright position to prevent contact with the stopper is recommended. It is best to use dark blue serum Trace Element/Trace Mineral tubes (*not* sodium citrate tubes, which are also blue but are designed for coagulation assays and are not valid for trace mineral analysis).[31] Trace Mineral/Trace Element tubes should be labeled as such (**Fig. 1**).

PESTICIDES
Herbicides

Herbicides are pesticides designed to target unwanted vegetation and currently available products are considered to be relatively safe to horses and other mammals. There are numerous classes of herbicides. Many older herbicides with significant negative health effects (eg, arsenicals) are no longer available. However, animals may be exposed to old stores of such compounds.[32] Although occurrences are possible year-round, intoxications are likely to be seasonal during the spring and fall when these compounds are applied to either prevent growth of weeds or as defoliates. Ultimately, there is less information regarding the effects of the majority of herbicides on horses with the exception of a select few compounds.[33] Arsenicals (monosodium methyl arsenate) and dipyridyl (paraquat and diquat) herbicides still pose significant health concern to horses if consumed.[34] Currently, there is no evidence that glyphosate (Roundup), when used correctly and at labeled concentrations, causes adverse health effects in animals and is unlikely to cause clinical issues in horses.[35]

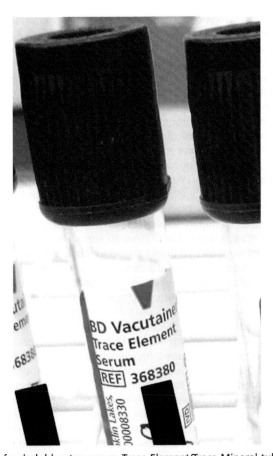

Fig. 1. Example of a dark blue-top serum Trace Element/Trace Mineral tube.

Sources include improperly stored concentrates, forages to which products have recently been applied, and access to old products.[32] The most likely source is the consumption of forages following turn out to pasture where herbicides have been applied and the graze-out period has not been met.[34,36]

Similar to fertilizers, the mechanisms of action of herbicides depend on the compound. All can cause direct irritation to the skin, mucosal membranes, and GI tract. Clinical signs also largely depend on the specific compound and the concentration. GI discomfort/colic is the only clinical sign occurring with exposure to most current herbicides. More severe GI issues are expected following the consumption of arsenical herbicides including necrosis and sloughing leading to hemorrhagic diarrhea. Signs are akin to those of arsenical insecticides.[20] Consumption of paraquat or recently applied forages may result in seizures and recumbency as well as progressive respiratory failure.[34] Oral mucous membranes may become inflamed and sensitive.[36] Both arsenical and dipyridyl herbicides also have the potential to cause renal complications.[34]

Death is unlikely following ingestion of most modern herbicides and associated sprayed forages. Lesions associated with arsenical products include GI necrosis and hemorrhage.[20] Severe pulmonary edema, necrosis, and fibrosis are expected following paraquat ingestion.[34] Diagnosis is primarily made by history of exposure to herbicide compounds and corresponding signs and lesions. Urine serves an ideal sample for herbicide testing because many compounds are excreted unmetabolized. Fresh and formalin-fixed lung should be submitted for the determination of paraquat as the compound concentrates in the lung tissues. Paraquat may also be detected in liver and kidney.[34] Fresh liver and kidney, as well as formalin-fixed GI tract, are useful in diagnosing arsenical herbicide poisoning.[20,34] See also the "Metals" section.

Treatment is supportive. Antioxidant therapy may be initiated following paraquat exposure.[34] Bentonite Fullers Earth can be used to treat for paraquat.[37] Ultimately, the prognosis is poor in individuals that consume arsenical or paraquat herbicides. Dimercaprol can be used to treat As poisoning.[22]

Insecticides

Organophosphates/Carbamates

Organophosphates (OPs) and carbamates are both cholinesterase inhibitors, and are often considered together. There are numerous products used in industry, agriculture, and residential settings. Common sources include baits, pour-on applications, and treated seeds. Inadvertent addition of such compounds to rations and consumption of treated or bait products serve as likely sources for equine poisonings.[38] Both are neurotoxic and exert their effects through the inhibition of acetylcholinesterase (AChE).[39] Inhibition of this enzyme results in a reduced capacity to break down acetylcholine in the synapse, leading to continuous stimulation of both muscarinic and nicotinic receptors. OPs covalently bind AChE with the bond potentially permanent through aging. Conversely, carbamates may spontaneously separate from AChE.[39,40]

Onset of clinical signs often occurs soon after ingestion or exposure to these compounds due to rapid absorption and distribution throughout the body. The severity and duration of signs are dose dependent. However, it is often difficult to ascertain the dose received. Certain pharmaceuticals, such as phenothiazines and aminoglycosides, may exacerbate intoxications and should be avoided.[41]

Clinical signs associated with OPs and carbamates include muscarinic and nicotinic signs. Overstimulation of muscarinic cholinergic receptors results in parasympathetic signs including excessive salivation, lacrimation, urination, and defecation.[40,42] Affected individuals may also experience GI complications, bradycardia, miosis, and dyspnea.[43] Stimulation of nicotinic receptors may result in uncontrollable tremors, muscle fasciculations, and paralysis. Death results from extreme bronchoconstriction and decreased functionality of respiratory muscles.[40] Not all cases present in the same manner as described. In some instances, CNS overstimulation may supersede the clinical presentation described above and instead result in seizures from CNS malfunction, tachycardia, and mydriasis.[44] It is important not to dismiss OPs and carbamates as possible causes for intoxication even if an animal is not exhibiting parasympathetic signs.

OP/carbamate poisonings in equine can be challenging to diagnose. Neither gross nor microscopic lesions are typically present.[43] Diagnosis depends on clinical signs, history of exposure, and supporting analytical evidence. Submission of whole blood, fresh brain, liver, GI contents, and suspect material should be considered in cases of suspected intoxication. AChE activity can be measured in the brain (postmortem) and whole blood (antemortem). Inhibition of AChE in brain or blood greater than 50% indicates exposure and is consistent with poisoning. Activity levels of AChE less than 25% are definitive for intoxication. Practitioners should be aware that carbamates may spontaneously release from AChE even after sample collection. Therefore, measured AChE activity may be normal even if in a horse with toxicosis.[45,46] It is important to note that select products approved for use in equines may reduce AChE activity, so a complete history is important in order to differentiate. Fresh tissue and GI content can be analyzed to determine the specific compound.[43]

Atropine is an antidote for OP/carbamate poisonings. Atropine sulfate can be given 0.1 to 0.2 mg/kg with one-fourth of the dose going IV and the remaining given intramuscular.[47] Administration of this compound controls the effects associated with muscarinic receptors but not those associated nicotinic receptors. Caution should be used when administering atropine to horses as excess can cause GI stasis. When it is unclear whether a cholinesterase inhibitor is the problem, administration of a 0.02 mg/kg atropine test dose can be provided IV to evaluate for response.[47] An alternative treatment, although expensive in a horse, is pralidoxime chloride (2-PAM) that breaks the bond between AChE and OPs. This compound can be a good addition to the treatment of OPs with atropine because it aids in controlling nicotinic symptoms. The recommended dose of 2-PAM for horses is 20 mg/kg slowly IV and can be repeated every 4 to 6 hours as needed.[40,47] The use of 2-PAM for carbamates has less effect due to spontaneous separation from AChE. Antidotes for OP poisonings gradually become less effective over time because the bond between OP and AChE gets stronger.

Pyrethroids
Pyrethroid insecticides are the synthetic analogs of pyrethrins produced by select flora. There are many pyrethroid products designed for use in horses. Intoxications do occur following excessive application of approved products or ingestion of concentrates.[48] These compounds are a significant source of poisonings in horses.[33] Most products are designed for dermal application but intoxications can happen through accidental ingestion or inhalation. Dermal absorption in the horse is slow with less than 2% accumulated by the body. Absorption through ingestion or inhalation can result in more rapid and greater absorption. Overdoses result in hyperexcitability due to impaired sodium ion channels.[49,50] Slowed closing of these channels allows for extended depolarization and lowering of action potential.

Clinically, symptoms of pyrethroid overdose in equines may closely resemble OP/carbamate poisoning. Individuals may exhibit increase salivation, be hyperexcitable, tremors, and seizures. Differentiation can be aided through failure of treatment of OP with atropine.[47] No specific antidote is available for pyrethroid intoxication, so supportive care through relieving respiratory distress, minimizing seizure activity, and maintaining hydration is critical.[48] Bathing individuals with water and dish washing detergent following dermal exposure aides in decontamination.[48,51]

PROPYLENE GLYCOL

PG is a colorless, odorless compound found in select antifreeze products and is also commonly used to treat ketosis in cattle. Despite antifreeze products, in which PG is advertised to be safe for pets, the compound is toxic to horses at 6 mL/kg body weight (BW).[13] The most common circumstance of poisoning in horses is accidental administration of PG mistaken for mineral oil. Such poisonings are likely to occur due to the similar packaging, labeling, and physical appearance. Multiple reports of such events are reported in the literature.[12,13,52]

PG is thought to exert its toxic effects in a similar fashion to that of ethanol through the increase of D-lactate within nervous tissue resulting in CNS depression.[53] The clinical presentation of PG poisoning may present identical to that of both ethanol and early EG. Onset of clinical signs may occur within as little as 15 minutes and include ataxia, salivation, sweating, and abdominal pain.[12,52] When consumed at high concentrations, the breath and feces may become malodorous.[13] Within 24 hours, individuals may develop labored breathing. Lateral recumbency and death are noted to occur when PG is provided at 16.7 mL/kg.[12]

As with EG poisoning, urine and serum can both be used to test for the presence of PG. Bloodwork often reveals acidosis with an increased anion gap. Due to the similar clinical presentation to that of both ethanol and early EG poisoning, as well as bloodwork indicative of acidosis, a complete and accurate history is critical in diagnosis and treating PG because the treatments between PG and EG differ.[12] Inappropriate diagnosis of EG instead of PG poisoning may lead to no response to treatment and potential iatrogenic ethanol poisoning. Successful treatment of PG intoxication has reportedly consisted of intravenous administration of a combination of sodium bicarbonate (1 L), dexamethasone (60 mL), and 1250 mL vitamin C. Sodium bicarbonate and vitamin C administration were repeated every 2 hours over 10 hours and every 4 hours over 12 hours respectively. In addition to the initial treatment, continuous administration of LRS at 8 mL/kg/h is also suggested.[13] The use of vitamin C was to aid in the reduction of any oxidative damage. Activated charcoal has been used following gastric lavage. If treatment is started early enough, horses may recover in as little as 4 hours. However, practitioners and owners should be aware that, following recovery, the malodorous breath and feces may remain for a period of time in exposed individuals.

CLINICS CARE POINTS

- Although exposure to many agricultural and industrials toxins is common, occurrence of intoxications with these agents is relatively uncommon.
- Most modern herbicides and fertilizers are unlikely to cause significant health complications in horses.
- Clinical signs in horses vary greatly depending on the agricultural or industrial toxin involved.
- While antidotes are available for several toxins, many agents require supportive care.

DISCLOSURE

The authors declare no potential commercial or financial conflicts of interest with respect to research, authorship, and/or this publication.

REFERENCES

1. Carson TL. Chapter 20: Household and Industrial Products, In: Plumlee K.H. In: *Clinical veterinary toxicology.* St. Louis, MO: Mosby; 2004. p. 139–76.
2. Morgan S. Ammonia pipeline rupture: risk assessment to cattle. Vet Hum Toxicol 1997;39(3):159–61.
3. Fitzgerald SD, Grooms DL, Scott M, et al. Acute anhydrous ammonia intoxication in cattle. J Vet Diagn Invest 2006;18(5):485–9.
4. Welch A. Exposing the dangers of anhydrous ammonia. Nurse Pract Am J Prim Health Care 2006;31(11):40–5.
5. Latenser BA, Lucktong TA. Anhydrous Ammonia Burns: Case Presentation and Literature Review. J Burn Care Rehabil 2000;21(1):40–2.
6. Beasley VR, Buck W. Acute ethylene glycol toxicosis: A review. Vet Hum Toxicol 1980;22(4):255–63.
7. Bischoff K. Chapter 72: Propylene Glycol. In: Peterson ME, Talcott PA, Small, editors. *animal toxicology.* 3rd edition. St. Louis, MO: W.B. Saunders; 2013. p. 763–7.
8. Swor TM, Aubry P, Murphey ED, et al. Acute ethylene glycol toxicosis in a horse. Equine Vet Educ 2002;14(5):234–9.
9. Fritz SA, Ensley SM, Njaa BL. Case report: Bovine ethylene glycol toxicosis. Bov Pract 2021;55(2):104–7.
10. Jacobsen D, McMartin KE. Methanol and ethylene glycol poisonings: mechanism of toxicity, clinical course, diagnosis and treatment. Med Toxicol 1986;1(5):309–34.
11. McQuade DJ, Dargan PI, Wood DM. Challenges in the diagnosis of ethylene glycol poisoning. Ann Clin Biochem 2014;51(2):167–78.
12. Dorman D, Haschek W. Fatal propylene glycol toxicosis in a horse. J Am Vet Med Assoc 1991;198(9):1643–4.
13. McClanahan S, Hunter J, Murphy M, et al. Propylene glycol toxicosis in a mare. Vet Hum Toxicol 1998;40(5):294–6.
14. Albretsen JC. Chapter 20: Household and Industrial Products, In: Plumlee K.H. In: *Clinical veterinary toxicology.* St. Louis, MO: Mosby; 2004. p. 139–76.
15. Osweiler GD, Carson TL, Buck WB, et al. Household and commercial products.. 3rd edition. Dubuque, IA: Kendall/Hunt Pub. Co; 1985. p. 381–9.
16. Villar D, Schwartz KJ, Carson TL, et al. Acute poisoning of cattle by fertilizer-contaminated water. Vet Hum Toxicol 2003;45(2):88–90.
17. Oruc HH, Akkoc A, Uzunoglu I, et al. Nitrate poisoning in horses associated with ingestion of forage and alfalfa. J Equine Vet Sci 2010;30(3):159–62.
18. Hintz H, Lowe J, Clifford A, et al. Ammonia intoxication resulting from urea ingestion by ponies. J Am Vet Med Assoc 1970;157:963–6.
19. Council NR. Mineral tolerance of animals. Washingon, DC: The National Academies Press; 2005.
20. Pace L, Turnquist S, Casteel S, et al. Acute arsenic toxicosis in five horses. J Veterinary Pathology 1997;34(2):160–4.
21. Puls RJBC, Canada. Mineral levels in animal health. Diagnostic data. Sherpa International, Clearbrook 1994;48.

22. Bertin F, Baseler L, Wilson C, et al. Arsenic Toxicosis in Cattle: Meta-Analysis of 156 Cases. J Vet Intern Med 2013;27(4):977–81.
23. Madejón P, Domínguez MT, Murillo J. Evaluation of pastures for horses grazing on soils polluted by trace elements. Ecotoxicology 2009;18:417–28.
24. Edens LM, Robertson J, Feldman B. Cholestatic hepatopathy, thrombocytopenia and lymphopenia associated with iron toxicity in a thoroughbred gelding. Equine Vet J 1993;25(1):81–4.
25. Ibrahim W, Lee U-S, Yeh C-C, et al. Oxidative stress and antioxidant status in mouse liver: effects of dietary lipid, vitamin E and iron. J Nutr 1997;127(7): 1401–6.
26. Palacios H, Iribarren I, Olalla M, et al. Lead poisoning of horses in the vicinity of a battery recycling plant. Sci Total Environ 2002;290(1–3):81–9.
27. Sojka JE, Hope W, Pearson D. Lead toxicosis in 2 horses: similarity to equine degenerative lower motor neuron disease. J Vet Intern Med 1996;10(6):420–3.
28. Allen K. Laryngeal paralysis secondary to lead toxicosis. Equine Vet Educ 2010; 22(4):182–6.
29. Bridges C, Moffitt P. Influence of variable content of dietary zinc on copper metabolism of weanling foals. Am J Vet Res 1990;51(2):275–80.
30. Hoyt J, Potter G, Greene L, et al. Copper balance in miniature horses fed varying amounts of zinc. J Equine Vet Sci 1995;15(8):357–9.
31. Dziwenka M. and Coppock R., Zinc, In: Plumlee K.H., *Clinical veterinary toxicology*, 2004, Mosby; St. Louis, MO, 193–230.
32. Caloni F, Cortinovis C, Rivolta M, et al. Suspected poisoning of domestic animals by pesticides. Sci Total Environ 2016;539:331–6.
33. Nagy A, Cortinovis C, Spicer L, et al. Long-established and emerging pesticide poisoning in horses. Equine Vet Educ 2019;31(9):496–500.
34. Padalino B, Bozzo G, Monaco D, et al. Avvelenamento da paraquat in cavalli da carne pugliesi. J Ippologia 2012;23(3):15–21.
35. Cortinovis C, Davanzo F, Rivolta M, et al. Glyphosate-surfactant herbicide poisoning in domestic animals: an epidemiological survey. Vet Rec 2015; 176(16):413.
36. Calderbank A, McKenna R, Stevens M, et al. Grazing trials on paraquat-treated pasture. J Sci Food Agric 1968;19(5):246–50.
37. Dasta JF. Paraquat poisoning: a review. Am J Health Syst Pharm 1978;35(11): 1368–72.
38. Plumlee KH, Richardson ER, Gardner IA, et al. Effect of time and storage temperature on cholinesterase activity in blood from normal and organophosphorus insecticide-treated horses. J Vet Diagn Invest 1994;6(2):247–9.
39. Fukuto TR. Mechanism of action of organophosphorus and carbamate insecticides. Environ Health Perspect 1990;87:245–54.
40. Fikes JD. Organophosphorus and carbamate insecticides. Veterinary Clinics of North America. Small Animal Practice 1990;2:353–67.
41. Sidell FR. Soman and sarin: clinical manifestations and treatment of accident of accidental poisoning by organophosphates. Clin Toxicol 1974;7(1):1–17.
42. Krieger R, South P, Flores I, et al. Toxicity of methomyl following intravenous administration in the horse. Vet Hum Toxicol 1998;40(5):267–9.
43. Meerdink C. Organophosphorus and carbamate insecticide poisoning in large animals. Veterinary Clinics of North America. Food Animal Practice 1989;2: 375–89.
44. Tafuri J, Roberts J. Organophosphate poisoning. Ann Emerg Med 1987;16(2): 193–202.

45. Risher JF, Mink FL, Stara JF. The toxicologic effects of the carbamate insecticide aldicarb in mammals: a review. Environ Health Perspect 1987;72:267–81.

46. Plumlee KH, Tor ER. Total cholinesterase activity in discrete brain regions and retina of normal horses. J Vet Diagn Invest 1997;9(1):109–10.

47. Muhammad G, Rashid I, Firyal S. Practical aspects of treatment of organophosphate and carbamate insecticide poisoning in animals. Matrix Sci Pharma 2017; 1(1):10–1.

48. Anadón A, Martínez-Larrañaga M, Martínez M. Use and abuse of pyrethrins and synthetic pyrethroids in veterinary medicine. Vet J 2009;182(1):7–20.

49. Bradbury SP, Coats JR. Comparative toxicology of the pyrethroid insecticides. Rev Environ Contam Toxicol 1989;133–77.

50. Ray DE, Ray D, Forshaw PJ. Pyrethroid insecticides: poisoning syndromes, synergies, and therapy. J Toxicol Clin Toxicol 2000;38(2):95–101.

51. Tucker SB, Flannigan SA, Ross C. Inhibition of cutaneous paresthesia resulting from synthetic pyrethroid exposure. Int J Dermatol 1984;23(10):686–9.

52. Van den Wollenberg L, Pellicaan C, Müller K. Intoxication with propylene glycol in two horses. Tijdschr Diergeneeskd 2000;125(17):519–23.

53. Christopher M, Eckfeldt J, Eaton J. Propylene glycol ingestion causes D-lactic acidosis. Laboratory Investigation Journal of Technical Methods Pathology 1990;62(1):114–8.

Moving?

Make sure your subscription moves with you!

To notify us of your new address, find your **Clinics Account Number** (located on your mailing label above your name), and contact customer service at:

Email: journalscustomerservice-usa@elsevier.com

800-654-2452 (subscribers in the U.S. & Canada)
314-447-8871 (subscribers outside of the U.S. & Canada)

Fax number: 314-447-8029

Elsevier Health Sciences Division
Subscription Customer Service
3251 Riverport Lane
Maryland Heights, MO 63043

*To ensure uninterrupted delivery of your subscription, please notify us at least 4 weeks in advance of move.

Printed and bound by CPI Group (UK) Ltd, Croydon, CR0 4YY

03/10/2024

01040470-0018